THE INCREDIBLE SHRINKING BRAIN

THE
Incredible
Shrinking
BRAIN

STEFAN LERNER, MD

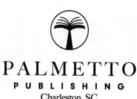

PALMETTO

P U B L I S H I N G

Charleston, SC

www.PalmettoPublishing.com

Hardcover ISBN: 979-8-8229-2605-9
Paperback ISBN: 979-8-8229-2606-6

The Terrible Shrinking Brain

How hyperapoptosis causes the premature death of countless neurons (brain cells) not only in neurological illnesses such as stroke, multiple sclerosis, and Parkinson's disease

But Also
In so-called "mental" illnesses like schizophrenia, bipolar disorder, and severe major depression.
Question:
Are so-called "mental" illnesses really "mental?" Or should that stigmatizing, belittling frame of reference be discarded? (But psychiatry will never do it.)
Stefan Lerner, M.D.

Major Depression, Bipolar Disorder, Schizophrenia

People with these illnesses are *not* "mentally" ill. They are *not* "mental cases." They have neurological-like *physical* brain disorders paralleling physical neurological illnesses.

Author's Note

The mission of this book is to promote radical change in the so-called field of mental health. In the process, it is highly critical of the psychiatric profession as a whole while acknowledging that some psychiatrists maintain high standards of care. If your own psychiatrist has been helpful to you, by all means, continue treatment with that doctor. If not, an excellent second opinion is probably available at a teaching hospital that has a direct association with a school of medicine. The psychiatric attendings in these institutions generally maintain high standards of care. There is one such center in most states.

Contents

Introduction

This book has been written with two audiences in mind, first, psychiatrists, and second the general public.

For Psychiatrists:

Dr. Thomas Insel, M.D., Senior Psychiatrist and former Director of the NIMH, resigned that position to conduct an extensive survey of outcomes for treatments of mental illnesses in the United States. His assessments and conclusions are published in his 2022 book, "Healing Our Path From Mental Illness to Mental Health." According to one reviewer, it is "A bold, expert and actionable map for America's broken mental health care system." Dr. Insel offers a comprehensive plan for our failing system, and for families trying to discern their way forward.

His ultimate conclusion about the collective outcome of results of treatment, Net Zero!

(Although, of course, some fortunate clients and patients do benefit.)

Psychiatry is an important element of the mental health care system, of course. What is its role in the overall dismal results of the mental health system? This book focuses more specifically on psychiatry. How can the specialty collectively improve outcomes?

Neuroscience and imaging studies have established the relevance of aberrant apoptosis - (hyperapoptosis) - as an important pathophysiological process in major depression, bipolar disorder and schizophrenia, but there is little attention paid to it in the psychiatric literature. It is now known accelerated loss of neurons leads to decrements in the volume of brain tissue, observable in imaging studies at least in series! One logical conclusion might be there should be a further emphasis on pharmacological treatments, that is promoting expertise in clinical psychopharmacology and promoting it as a medical specialty in its own right.

Lithium is seriously under-prescribed by psychiatrists in the United States, which may contribute to poor outcomes. Dr. Robert M. Post, MD reviews the therapeutic benefits of this molecule. There is on-going attention to it in this book. In the last chapter it is inquired what psychiatry can do to improve outcomes. Nine suggestions are given.

Most importantly, a fundamental issue is discussed, the very negative aspects of continuing the entire "mental" illness classification. As we proceed into the twenty-first century, is this how we wish to continue to categorize these illnesses? One option could be to re-identify them with the same "neuro" root as in neurology, "neuriatric," as well to designate the many disorders in the DSM not as "mental" disorders, but as cognitive, emotional, behavioral and personality dysregulations.

For the public, those interested in "mental" health:

Marilyn Monroe, Carrie Fisher and Anthony Bourdain were remarkable people, colorful, so creative, so accomplished. Enjoy their stories. Yet, they all had the same ending, death by suicide. How could that happen to them? (And if it happened to them, how about us average individuals?) They never had the luck and good fortune to be treated by a truly competent psychiatrist. Indeed, they would not know what a truly competent psychiatrist was, even if they fell over one. It's Russian Roulette! So, one purpose of this book is to learn what psychiatric competence is and how to locate such practitioners.

There is much technical information in the book which is meant for the psychiatrists to review. Even lay-people can just momentarily scan some of the material which demonstrate the basic driving pathological causes of so-called "mental" illnesses are PHYSICAL dysregulations. In other words, they are really physical brain illnesses not "mental" ones. And, of course, the "mental" label is burdened by stigma which alienates many prospective patients. The entire categorization of "mental" illness needs to be erased, and a physical identity instead established. For example, a tentative relabeling could be "neuriatric" illnesses, using the same root, "neuro," as in neurological illnesses. This may turn off prospective patients less than being labeled a "mental case." Between 50-60% of prospective patients avoid "mental" health treatment currently, being "gun-shy" of the "mental" health care system. That really contributes to the poor outcomes of treatments (and lack thereof), Dr. Innes has so clearly outlined.

There are a number of sections the lay-person might just scan or skip, but try to read about HYPERAPOPTOSIS, just to catch the "flavor" of the complex PHYSICAL etiologies of major depression, bipolar disorder and schizophrenia. (Not an Oedipus complex is mentioned.) Don't expect to know the meaning of most of the material, they are PHYSICAL causes, most certainly not "MENTAL ONES!"

May Be Scanned or Skipped

- Imaging Studies. Summary studies in M.D.D.
- Imaging Studies before and after ECT
- Bipolar Disorder, Multiple Physical Dysregulations in the brain
- Bipolar disorder and Neuroscience (not Psychiatry)
- Changes in Ventricular size and Cerebral Gray matter.
- Physiological Function of the Brain Networks in Bipolar Disorder
- Prefrontal Cortical Abnormalities in Bipolar Disorder
- Imaging Differences Between Bipolar and Unipolar Disorder
- Additional Research Findings in Bipolar Disorder
- Changes in Neurophasticity and Neurotropin
- Changes in Intracellular Signaling Cascades
- Schizophrenia
- Epilepsy
- Anomalous Brain Patterns in Major Psychiatric Disorders
- Quality of Life in Individuals: World Psychiatry

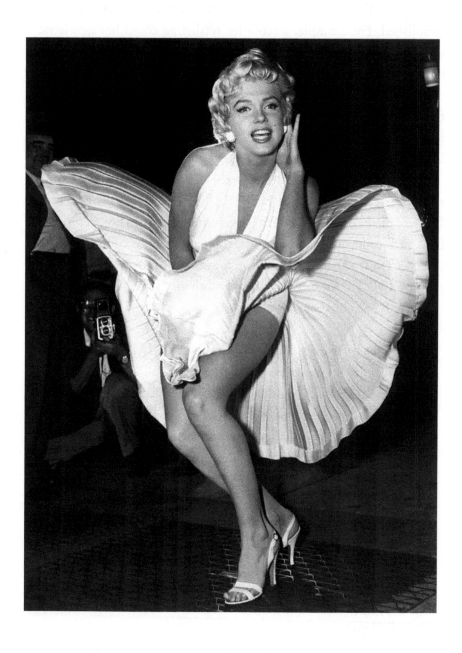

Marilyn Monroe

She died in her own home, which she had tastefully furnished, at 12305 Fifth Helena Drive in the Brentwood neighborhood of Los Angeles.[1] Her housekeeper, Eunice Murray, who lived with her, awoke at 3:00 a.m. on August 4, 1962, and noticed that the light under the door of Marilyn's room was still on. She went to check, but there was no reply. The door was locked. She next called Marilyn's psychiatrist, Dr. Ralph Greenson, who arrived at the house and broke into the bedroom through a window, finding Marilyn dead in her bed. Her physician arrived next, at around 3:50 a.m. He pronounced her dead. The Los Angeles Police Department was notified at 4:25 a.m. Marilyn was dead at age thirty-six, and there was an emptied bottle of barbiturate tablets on her nightstand. Her great ambition to be a serious, respected actress, toward which she studied and worked so diligently, evaporated. She deserved to become a great actress on stage and screen. She and her public would never be able to witness what could have been.

But they did get a "taste."

Legacy

In the sixty-plus years since her death, she has not been forgotten. According to *The Guide to United States Popular Culture*,[2] she remains an icon of that culture. A prominent historian, Gail Levin,

---

1   Marilyn Monroe. Wikipedia
2   The Guide to United States Popular Culture. June 15, 2001. Ray B. Browne (Editor), Pat Browne (Editor).

observed that Monroe may have been the most photographed person of the twentieth century. The American Film Institute named her the sixth-greatest female screen legend in American film history. The Smithsonian Institution has categorized her one of the one hundred most significant Americans of all time. *Variety* placed her in the top ten rankings of the greatest popular culture icons of the twentieth century. Hundreds of books have been written about her, and she has been featured in numerous films, plays, operas, and songs. Sixty years after her death, she also remains a valuable brand. Her name and image have been licensed for hundreds of products, including Max Factor, Chanel, Mercedes-Benz, and Absolut Vodka. Although there were critics of her acting ability, they were outnumbered by her boosters. Well-known critic Peter Bradshaw wrote that Monroe was a talented comedian who understood how comedy achieved its effects. Another prominent critic of the era, Roger Ebert, wrote that Monroe's eccentricities and neuroses on sets became notorious, but studios put up with her long after any other actress would have been blackballed because what they got back on the screen was magical.

But her beginnings were not auspicious.

Her Formative Years

Her mother, Gladys Pearl Baker, twenty-six, brought her two-week old daughter, Norma Jeane Mortenson, to a foster home in Hawthorne, California, on June 13, 1926.[3] There was no evident father. When Marilyn was three, her mother came to the foster home in an agitated state, where she locked out the foster mom, then put Marilyn in a duffel bag and started to take her away. The foster mom, back in action, blocked Gladys. When Marilyn was seven, the foster mom decided it was time that Marilyn and Gladys should be reunited. Gladys, at first, rose to the occasion, taking out a loan to buy a small house. But then things went awry for Gladys. At about the same time, her thirteen-year-old son, who had been taken from Gladys at birth by the father,

---

3   https://wwwbiography.com/news/marilyn-monroe-mother-relationship. pg. 1.

died; her grandfather hung himself, and she was laid off from her job at a Hollywood studio. Her response was to lash out at Marilyn. A year later, in 1934, her mother became extremely agitated in Marilyn's presence, requiring the police to appear. Gladys was diagnosed as a paranoid schizophrenic and hospitalized in a state psychiatric hospital. Marilyn was placed in a series of foster homes, perhaps twelve in all, and also spent time in an orphanage. There is a strong likelihood that she was sexually abused more than once: by a cousin, by the boyfriend of an acquaintance, and by a foster parent. Marilyn last saw her mother in 1962, when she was attempting to get her to take her Thorazine medication. Her mother refused, insisting all she needed was prayer. Finally, when her mother started to depart, Marilyn slipped her a flask. And then a compliment: that Norma Jeane was a good girl.

Alexandra Kathryn Mosca, in her article "The Sad and Untimely Death of America's Fantasy,"[4] concluded that her fate was sealed at birth. She was born to a mentally unstable mother. There was no presence of a father. In her formative years, she lived through a succession of abusive foster homes. She was never able to find security and happiness and was preoccupied with death. She attributes a number of statements to Marilyn, although they appear without quotes, revealing a sense of doom: "I wonder why I go on, I feel miserable, I hate it, it hurts too much. Death has got to be better than this. I'd almost rather be crazy than feel this anxiety churning inside me. I'd rather be dead."

This author's comment: rather than reflecting a congenital sense of doom since birth, these statements are typical symptoms of clinical depression, which was never competently diagnosed or treated, evidently, throughout her life. Mosca expresses wonder that in spite of Marilyn's morbid perspective, she gained worldwide acclaim. In her sixteen-year career, she was in twenty-nine movies, with a "persona she had carefully constructed" that "deftly masked her tortured existence." This author does not believe she was in a permanent state of agony. She kept millions and millions entertained, made them laugh, amused

---

4   https://www.qcc.cuny.edu/socialscience/ppecorino/ss680/Funeral_Marilyn_Monroe.html

and aroused men, and charmed them all. It was not just a facade; her spirit showed through.

Her attraction to the movies started early. Some of her foster families would drop her off for the day at a cinema. "I'd sit all day and way into the night, up in the front. There was a screen so big and I, a kid all alone, and I loved it." (1), pg. 4. In 1942, her foster parents at the time had to relocate to West Virginia. California's child protection laws did not allow them to take Marilyn out of the state, and she was faced with having to return to the orphanage. To avoid this, she made a decision to marry her next-door neighbor, a factory worker, James Dougherty. She was unhappy in the marriage. In April 1944, when he was shipped out to the Pacific as a serviceman during World War II, she began to work in a munitions factory in Van Nuys, California. It was there that a United States Army Air Forces photographer noticed her and photographed her for his project of shooting morale-boosting pictures of female workers. Hence, she began a modeling career. The owner of the agency where she worked found her to be one of its most ambitious and hardworking models. Marilyn's photographs appeared on numerous magazine covers of the era, thirty-three at least. Also, the owner facilitated Marilyn's enrollment in an acting agency. She obtained a six-month contract at 20th Century Fox. She also formally adopted the stage name "Marilyn Monroe." At Fox, she spent the six months learning acting, singing, and dancing and observing the filmmaking process. She had her first film roles in bit parts. As she later commented, it was her first taste of what real acting in a real drama could be, and she was hooked. Some of her teachers, however, were not confident about her potential, thinking she was too shy and insecure to have a future in acting. Fox did not renew her contract, and she returned to modeling, but she did not give up on succeeding as an actress. She took the initiative, frequenting producers' offices, befriending them, and entertaining influential male guests at studio functions. A friend, Joseph M. Schenck, a studio executive, introduced her to the head of Columbia Pictures, Harry Cohn. At Columbia, her hair was bleached blonde, and her look was modeled

THE INCREDIBLE SHRINKING BRAIN

after Rita Hayworth's. She played in a low-budget musical, *Ladies of the Chorus* (1948), but her contract was not renewed. Subsequently, she met the vice president of the William Morris Agency, Johnny Hyde. He played a very strategic role in her life. He arranged for her to act in several films; of particular note were *All About Eve* (1950) and *The Asphalt Jungle* (1950) (ibid, pg. 6). Even though her appearances had been brief, she was noticed by some important persons in the industry. For example, 20th Century Fox gave her a seven-year contract, negotiated by Mr. Hyde, but then he died of a heart attack, devastating Marilyn. Next, she appeared in three successful comedies. She was praised by critics, one describing her acting as superb. Another commented that she was one of the brightest up-and-coming actresses. Her popularity was growing. She was receiving several thousand fan letters a week, and she was dating prominent men such as actors Yul Brynner and Peter Lawford.

In March 1952, she was called to account by the studio administrators after they had learned that she had posed nude for a calendar in 1949. She handled the issue in a straightforward manner, explaining that she had been broke, desperate for money. Her public sympathized with her, and the publicity had a positive effect. She was featured on the cover of *Life* magazine, and the gossip columnist Hedda Hopper identified her as the talk of Hollywood, the cheesecake queen turned box office smash. In one movie starring Barbara Stanwyck, *Clash By Night*, she played a fish-cannery worker. To prepare, she spent time in a fish cannery. She obviously extended herself to give a good performance! *Variety*, writing about her, commented, "She has an ease of delivery which makes her a cinch for popularity." She made two other films in 1952, the comedies *We're Not Married* and *Monkey Business*. She burnished her image as a sex symbol by wearing a revealing dress when she was the Grand Marshal at the Miss America Pageant parade, and she told gossip columnist Earl Wilson that she usually wore no underwear. To alleviate symptoms of anxiety and insomnia, she had started to take sleeping pills and barbiturates. She had become severely addicted by 1956. When the movie *Niagara* was released in

1953, women's clubs criticized it as immoral, but *The New York Times* commented that *Niagara Falls* and Miss Monroe were something to see, that she could be seductive even when she walked. In her second film of 1953, *Gentlemen Prefer Blondes*, her screen persona as a "dumb blonde" firmly caught on. Her presentation of the song "Diamonds Are a Girl's Best Friend" was considered to be a gem! In *How to Marry a Millionaire*, released in November 1953, she played a naïve model who, along with her friends, played by Betty Grable and Lauren Bacall, strategized to find rich men to marry. In December 1953, in the first issue of *Playboy*, publisher Hugh Hefner featured a nude photograph of Marilyn without her permission.

By the mid-1950s, Marilyn was one of 20th Century Fox's most popular actresses, but the studio head, one Darryl F. Zanuck, had taken an early dislike for Marilyn, and compared to actors and actresses of equal stature, she was considerably underpaid and had little say in the production of her movies. In January 1954, she put her foot down, refusing to begin shooting another musical comedy, *The Girl in Pink Tights*. Even that situation became front-page news. That same month, she and the famous, retired baseball star Joe DiMaggio were married. He, of course, was the renowned slugger and center fielder for the New York Yankees, nicknamed the "Yankee Clipper" or "Joltin' Joe," from 1938-1942 and 1946-1951. (If you happen to own mint baseball cards from his early career, you're in luck: prices range from $75,000 to $200,000.) DiMaggio had business in Tokyo and suggested that they both go for their honeymoon, with the added benefit of Marilyn taking a break from the conflict with Zanuck and the studio. She made a side trip to Korea and participated in the United Service Organizations, singing for sixty thousand marines over four days. Finally, Fox settled with her, promising a new contract and a bonus of $100,000 (perhaps approximately nearly $2 million in 2022 dollars).

In September 1954, she played in Billy Wilder's comedy *The Seven Year Itch*. The studio arranged for a publicity stunt by posing Marilyn in an ornate white dress over a subway grating. The photograph captured her with her dress blown up, exposing her legs as a subway train passed below. The "subway-grate scene" became world-famous. However, her husband, Joe DiMaggio, strongly disapproved of the scene, resulting in a final breach of the marital bond. Marilyn got a Mexican divorce soon after, ending a nine-month marriage. There were intimations that he was controlling, jealous, and possibly physically abusive. Marilyn moved to New York in 1955, spending the year studying acting and attending the Actors Studio run by Lee Strasberg. He and his wife befriended her as if she were a member of the family.

Even after they divorced, she and DiMaggio remained friends. She dated an array of famous men: Marlon Brando, Frank Sinatra, and the playwright Arthur Miller. Her studio raised concerns about her budding relationship with Miller, as he was being investigated by the FBI and had been subpoenaed by the House Un-American Activities Committee. She, however, was not to be instructed about with whom she could have a relationship. The FBI did open a file on her.

Evidently, Fox wanted Marilyn more than she wanted Fox. They gave her a contract in which she would make four films for a salary of $400,000 (probably $7-8 million in 1922 dollars), and she was given production rights to choose her own producer, director, and cinematographers.

There was additional criticism of her relationship with Miller by some journalists. Walter Winchell, the prominent gossip columnist and radio host, commented that America's best-known blond moving-picture star had become the darling of the left-wing intelligentsia. *Variety* pithily reported, "Egghead weds hourglass."

In 1956, she played Cherie, a saloon singer whose dreams are complicated by a naïve cowboy, in the drama *Bus Stop*. The noted Broadway director Joshua Logan, who at first had low expectations of her ability, ended up as a solid fan, comparing her to Charlie Chaplin in her ability to blend comedy and tragedy. The movie was released in August 1956. *The Saturday Review of Literature* commented that Monroe's performance dispelled once and for all the notion that she was merely a glamorous personality. Another prominent critic, Bosley Crowther, stated that viewers should hold on to their chairs and get set for a rattling surprise. Marilyn Monroe had finally proved herself an actress. She was nominated for the Golden Globe Award for Best Actress for her performance in *Bus Stop*.

In 1958, she had an ectopic pregnancy and a miscarriage. She was hospitalized for a barbiturate overdose, consistent with a developing barbiturate addiction.

But she could still perform at that juncture. In 1958, she costarred with Jack Lemmon and Tony Curtis in the film *Some Like It Hot*. She was induced to play another "dumb blonde," Sugar Kane, after she was promised 10 percent of the film's profits in addition to her salary. The film's production was notoriously difficult, with Marilyn obsessively demanding retakes and forgetting her lines. Tony Curtis said that kissing Marilyn was like kissing Hitler because there were so many retakes. Marilyn herself had a dejected opinion of the completed film, saying the production was like a sinking ship. Billy Wilder, the eminent director, however, had a different opinion: that anyone can remember lines, but it takes a real *artist* to come onto the set and not know her lines yet give the performance she did.

In spite of Marilyn's discouragement about *Some Like It Hot*, she earned a Golden Globe Award for Best Actress. Variety described her as a comedienne with that combination of sex appeal and timing that just can't be beat. Polls by the BBC voted it one of the best films ever made. Similar accolades were voiced by the American Film Institute and *Sight and Sound* magazine.

The last film she completed, *The Misfits*, directed by John Huston, also costarred Clark Gable, Eli Wallach, and Montgomery Clift. Her then-husband, Arthur Miller, had written the script. Marilyn, however, disliked the characterization Miller had written for her role in the film. They were at odds. He began an affair. She obtained a Mexican divorce. Unfortunately, her untreated barbiturate addiction had become so severe that her makeup could be properly applied only when she was sleeping. She again required hospitalization for detoxification. Even with these complications, Huston stated that when she was acting, she was not pretending to have an emotion; it was the real thing. She would go deep down within herself, find it, and bring it up into consciousness. The reviews of *The Misfits* were mixed. *Variety* found the character development choppy. The prominent movie critic Bosley Crowther found Monroe's role to be completely blank and unfathomable. More recently, however, some opinions have been far more favorable. Geoff Andrew of the British Film Institute called it a classic. Tony Tracy, a student of director Huston, registered her role as the most mature interpretation of her career. Geoffrey Macnab, the movie critic for *The Independent*, found her portrayal of her character's power of empathy extraordinary.

Subsequently, unfortunately, she was hospitalized for "depression." She next began to play in a film for Fox, *Something's Got to Give*, costarring Dean Martin and Cyd Charisse. Before the shooting was to begin, Marilyn came down with severe sinusitis. Her physicians vouchsafed that she was too ill to work. Fox began shooting without her, alleging that she was faking it. Evidently, the film was not completed. Fox fired her, also suing her for $750,000. Fox began spreading negative publicity about her, saying that she was "mentally disturbed." But Fox again changed course, awarding her a new contract.

The White Dress

It was described as "one of the most iconic images of the 20th century."[5] The white dress appeared in the movie *The Seven Year Itch*, directed by Billy Wilder and released in 1955. Marilyn's character and her costar, Tom Ewell, had just left the Trans-Lux 52nd Street theater on Lexington Avenue in Manhattan, where they had viewed *The Creature from the Black Lagoon*. When Marilyn's character heard the sound of a passing subway train coming from the grate near her, she stationed herself directly above the grate, the rising wind from the train blowing

---

5   The White Dress of Marilyn Monroe. Wikipedia pg1.

her dress up as she struck a delightful pose. After Marilyn's death in 1962, William Travilla, the designer of the dress, kept it locked up. After his death in 1990, the actress Debbie Reynolds acquired it, placing it in the Hollywood Motion Pictures Museum.[6] In 2011, she decided to sell it at auction. The estimated value was $1-2 million, but it sold for $5.6 million.[7]

At the original shooting of the scene, her then-husband, Joe DiMaggio, the retired baseball star for the New York Yankees, found the exposure of his wife's legs very distasteful. But the scene and the dress took off on a fame trajectory of their own. The dress was portrayed in subsequent films *Tommy* (1975), *The Woman in Red* (1984), *Shrek 2* (2004), *Blades of Glory* (2007), and *The House Bunny* (2008). *Glamour* magazine classified the dress as "one of history's most famous dresses." A survey conducted by Cancer Research UK voted it number one of all time in iconic celebrity fashion moments.

The dress was bought by Gotta Have It Collectibles on November 17, 2016. It currently resides in Ripley's Believe It or Not Museum. The purchase price had been $4.8 million. It is the most expensive dress in the world.

Forever Marilyn[8]

The twenty-six-foot statue of Marilyn with her white dress blown up to her waist, as of 2021, is situated among palm trees in Palm Springs, California. The 34,000-pound statue, made of painted stainless steel and aluminum, has had a testy existence and done a good deal of traveling about. The sculptor, Seward Johnson, intended it as a tribute to Marilyn. The "model" was from her movie *The Seven Year Itch*, when her character stepped on a grating as a subway train passed underneath, resulting in an "instant blast" of air blowing up her white dress, exposing her legs as she struck a delightful pose.

---

6   ibid, pg2
7   ibid, pg2
8   https://en.wikipedia.org/wiki/ForeverMarilyn.

The statue, created in 2011, was first displayed in the Magnificent Mile section of Chicago until it was moved to Palm Springs, California. On March 27, 2014, after a farewell ceremony in Palm Springs, it was transported to the Grounds For Sculpture in Hamilton, New Jersey for a retrospective of Seward Johnson's statues. It was so popular that it was held over after the retrospective ended.

In 2016, it was shipped to the Australian city of Bendigo for the Bendigo Art Gallery's Marilyn Monroe exhibition. Again, recrossing the Pacific Ocean, it was transported across the United States to Stamford, Connecticut, for another exhibition honoring Seward Johnson. Thirty-six of his sculptures were placed at different locations downtown, and of course, "Forever Marilyn" was the highlight. The statue caused a stir in Stamford, with some critics complaining that she was "flashing her underwear" at the First Congregational Church.

Next, she was disassembled and stored at a New Jersey location until the good mayor of Palm Springs, California, Robert Moon, elected to have the statue returned to Palm Springs for permanent exhibition. It was resurrected and unveiled in April 2021. But not everyone was happy with that. Efforts were being made by critics in a suit to remove her.

Forever Marilyn in Australia and China

Bendigo is a city in Victoria, Australia, with a population of approximately 118,000. The residents call themselves "Bendigonians." Gold had been discovered there in 1851, transforming it from a "sheep station" to a boomtown.

The Bendigo Art Gallery's exhibition centered on Marilyn was described as a "blockbuster" (fn1).[9] Eighty-six thousand people attended the opening. Fire crews had washed "Forever Marilyn" before the opening of the exhibition, stopping traffic. That coincided with what would have been her ninetieth birthday. Tourism Minister John Eren stated, "We're really hoping the Marilyn exhibition will have a lot more people

---

9   "Marilyn Monroe exhibition a big splash for Bendigo tourism." Abc.net.au.

visiting this area." And it did, with the exhibition director, Ms. Quinlan, stating, "Some of the very busy, busy days, you cannot get a table for dinner." Local businesses were benefiting. Ms. Quinlan commented, "I think people will be a little teary when she goes."

An academic course featuring Marilyn was being offered at La Trobe University, coinciding with the exhibition: a fully accredited elective subject, "Exhibiting Culture: Marilyn." Dr. Sue Gillet, who taught the course, said she was interested in "exploring women's roles in cinema." She added, "Marilyn was such an interesting figure in where she fitted into popular culture and politics." Contrary to her screen persona, she was bright and "a canny businesswoman."

Students who were enrolled in the course had access to the Bendigo Gallery's Marilyn Monroe exhibition and the Murray Art Museum Albury's exhibition, "Marilyn: Celebrating an American Icon."

"Forever Marilyn" in Shanzhai, China[10]

She was even slightly taller than the "Forever Marilyn" in America, but she had a dark fate. Photographs from China showed a giant "Forever Marilyn" sculpture lying face down in a dump in Guigang, China. It was apparently a giant copy of Seward's original, probably also made out of stainless steel. According to a report by NBC, several Chinese artists made it over a two-year period. There were some very minor differences. The Chinese Marilyn's heels were sharper and thicker. Did the paramount leader of China, Xi Jinping, disapprove of her?

Some Like It Hot

The question is asked: Why has Billy Wilder's "glittering master-piece"[11] topped the BBC's 100 Greatest Comedies film poll? Nicholas Barber explains why. "Its cast excels. Tony Curtis is a terrific actor, Jack Lemmon a dexterous comedian, and to boot, it stars Hollywood's

---

10 Hyperallergic.com
11 Billy Wilder's glittering masterpiece has topped BBC Culture=100 greatest comedy poll. Nicholas Barber explains why. 22 August 2017. http:www.bbc.com/culture/article/20170817.

most radiant sex symbol, Marilyn Monroe." The film "glides from moment to moment with the elegance of an Olympic figure skater and is a riot of spills, thrills, laughs and games."

Curtis plays Joe, who will transition to Josephine. Lemmon plays Jerry, who will transition to Daphne. They start out in the movie as two musicians, a saxophonist and a bassist, respectively, scraping out a living in winery Chicago. But they are in the wrong place at the wrong time. They are witnesses to a gang's killing spree, and the gangsters spot them. They are marked men. They know Spats Colombo (played by George Raft) and his gang will be determined to permanently silence them. That's when they don their disguises to pass themselves off as members of a female jazz orchestra headed for Florida. Josephine and Daphne end up on a sleeper train sharing the car with Sweet Sue's Society Syncopaters. They both find Marilyn's character, Sugar Kane Kumulchek, the band's ukulele player and singer, incredibly attractive. Sugar Kane, of course, discloses her secret to them, believing that they're women: that she is going to Florida to try to seduce a millionaire. When they arrive at the Seminole Ritz Hotel, Curtis/Joe/Josephine hatches his plot. He outfits himself to pass himself off as Junior, an heir to the Shell Oil fortune. He then arranges to be spotted by Sugar Kane on the beach, and he speaks to her in his finest Cary Grant accent. To learn the outcome, watch the movie. Nicholas Barber, the movie critic, summarizes the movie: "It has so much warmth that it carries the viewer upwards like a hot-air balloon."

The two following reviews were more immediately written after the movie was released in 1959.

A.H. Weiler, writing in *The New York Times* on March 30, 1959, comments that the movie's originators "have come up with a rare rib-tickling lampoon." Both the management and viewers at Loew's State Theatre couldn't stop themselves from "chortling with glee." He commends the director, Mr. Wilder, who "was abetted by such equally proficient operatives as Marilyn Monroe, Jack Lemmon and Tony Curtis. The movie is as constantly busy as picnickers fighting off angry wasps." The actors "make their points with explosive effect." Miss Monroe, as the band's "somewhat simple singer-ukulele player, whose figure simply cannot be overlooked," makes a vital contribution to "this madcap romp." She sings, in a whispery voice, two old numbers, "Running Wild" and "I Wanna Be Loved by You," in a fashion "which is the epitome of a dumb blonde and a talented comedienne."

Robert Ebert,[12] a prominent film critic at the time *Some Like It Hot* was released, came right out with it: "What a work of art and nature is Marilyn Monroe." The movie itself will be "an enduring treasure of the movies, a film of inspiration and meticulous craft." And the movie's musical numbers stand out because Monroe "sells the lyrics" like Frank Sinatra. Her rendition of "I Wanna Be Loved by You" is as "mesmerizing and blatantly a sexual scene ever seen in the movies, in which nudity would add nothing. She wears a clinging see-through dress, gauze covering the slopes of her breasts, the neckline scooping to a censor's eyebrow north of trouble. To witness her in the scene is to understand why no other actor, male or female, has more sexual chemistry with the camera than Monroe." The studios "put up with her eccentricities and neurosis…because what they got back on the screen is magical." There were so many takes of the scene where Marilyn kisses Curtis that he complained that kissing her was like kissing Hitler. "You remember what Curtis said, but when you watch the scene, all you can think is that Hitler must have been a terrible kisser." And about Marilyn's performance, Ebert said, "It is an act of will to watch anyone else when she's on the screen."

And a very recent (2020) movie review of *Some Like It Hot*.[13] "We Still Like It Hot. Zowie! Our critics and readers pondered the silliness and semiotics of *Some Like It Hot* with Jack Lemmon, Marilyn Monroe and Tony Curtis, all in tresses and tottering heels." (The review was published sixty-one years after the movie's release). The authors relate a bit of movie lore: that Billy Wilder approached David O. Selznick, the prominent producer and studio executive, who had produced the honorable, great movie epic *Gone With the Wind* (1939), the highest-grossing film

12   https:www.rogerebert.com/reviews.Somelikeithot.1959.
13   https:/www.nytimes.com/2020/06/02/we still like it hot.A.O. Scott. And Manola Darais.

of all time adjusted for inflation. He sketched out the storyline for Selznick, who commented, "You're crazy. You mean, real machine guns and blood in a comedy? Total failure." A.O. Scott commented, "It's a complicated picture, bracingly ahead of its time in some ways." And about Marilyn, the movie "certainly uses her to generate erotic heat in that almost invisible Orry-Kelly gown." Sugar, Marilyn's character, is described as "more than eye candy." She does something quite sophisticated by transitioning from a sex object to the role of sexual predator by seducing Josephine/Tony Curtis. Her performance "works to perfection." Scott emphasizes that "it's crucial to see that she helped create this iconic blond bombshell called Marilyn Monroe." While watching the movie, it made Scott "laugh out loud as few others do—a feeling shared by most readers." About Marilyn's performance, he says that "Sugar is especially fascinating because she's hypersexualized, babyish, knowing, and innocent, and her innocence is also sincere and a deception." He summarizes, "The whole movie feels like it was directed inside gigantic quotation marks. It's a live action cartoon—with rat-a-tat guns and laughs and gargoyle villains right out of Dick Tracy." When he first watched it in the mid-eighties at the Castro Theatre in San Francisco, he said he "had never heard higher howls of laughter" from the audience.

A final comment about Marilyn's raw appeal was made by Jack Lemmon, telling Curtis *in Some Like It Hot*, "Look at that. Look at how she moves. Like Jell-O on springs. She must have some sort of built-in motor. I tell you, it's a whole different sex."

More About Marilyn, Relationships
(Some Possibly Apocryphal)

Albert Einstein. In the late 1940s, the actress Shelley Winters and Marilyn shared an apartment. In her autobiography, Winters said that Marilyn had told her she had a brief affair with the esteemed physicist Albert Einstein. An interchange between them: She asked Einstein, "Would it not be wonderful if we had a child with your brains and my beauty?" He replied, "Yes, but imagine a child with my beauty and your brains."[14]

Joe DiMaggio. He was an American hero, the great center fielder and slugger of the New York Yankees, a true cultural icon with the aliases "Joltin' Joe," "The Yankee Clipper," and "the Bronx Bomber." In 1952, he asked an acquaintance to arrange a dinner date with her. By then she had appeared in two films that came to his attention, *Monkey Business* and *Don't Bother to Knock*. It was a case of mutual attraction culminating in their marriage, but the marriage lasted only nine months before Marilyn filed for a Mexican divorce. Perhaps his concept of marriage did not provide for a wife spotlighted by barrages of publicity. There were intimations that he was overly possessive, jealous, and possibly even physically abusive toward her. But from his subsequent behavior in the year before her death and over the period after, it became obvious he still loved her. (One can wish that somehow, they could have maintained their marriage by establishing a workable understanding. Perhaps she would have survived, even becoming a beloved personage in her old age.) After her death, he made all the funeral arrangements. He arranged for roses to be delivered to her crypt three times a week for the next twenty years. His dying words were that he would see her again.

Hugh Hefner. He did not ask her permission when he placed a nude photograph of her in the centerfold of the first edition of his magazine, *Playboy*. It doesn't appear that they were acquaintances or friends. Yet he purchased a crypt adjacent to hers for $75,000 (perhaps worth up to $1 million in 2022 dollars). He died fifty-five years after she did, in 2017, and now lies next to her for all eternity.

Arthur Miller. He was her third husband, an established playwright. Earlier in his career, in 1949, his masterwork play, *Death of a Salesman*, opened in New York City. It won the Tony Award for Best Play and a Pulitzer Prize for Drama. It was adapted into a movie in 1951, appeared in several television versions, and has had additional revivals on Broadway.

14 Homolog.US.

Monroe and Miller collaborated on what was to be her last feature film, *The Misfits*, he writes the part she was to play in it. She was very unhappy with his interpretation, feeling it emphasized certain negative aspects of herself. There arose, evidently, an unbridgeable disagreement, which may have been a factor in the dissolution of their marriage. A costar was Clark Gable, who also died within two years after the film was completed, at age fifty-nine.

Critique of *The Misfits*

Rotten Tomatoes.[15] This site lists thirty-one reviews of *The Misfits*. Three of them:

Kate Cameron, January 18, 2018, *New York Daily News*. She commented, "Gable has never done anything better on the screen, nor has Miss Monroe." She continued, "I believe it has a finer quality of and a greater dramatic interest, than any American product released last year."

Tim Brayton, Antagony and Ecstasy: "…such a fantastic acting showcase…" (August 3, 2012). He notes, however, that during the filming, Monroe was "deep in the throes of substance addiction." He summarized that *The Misfits* certainly "is not a terribly fun movie to watch, but it sure is a hell of an intense ride."

Beauty Icon.[16] "Legendary Hollywood goddess Marilyn Monroe is the most searched for name on the internet for beauty inspiration, according to a study, 'Recreate Yourself.'" Marilyn had 191,00 searches. Second was the famous model Twiggy, with 165,000. Third was a male model from England, David Bowie, with 150,000.

Her Impersonators

Marilyn still provides employment opportunities to talented young women six decades after her death. Michelle M.[17], a singer/actress/celebrity impersonator, has been performing in her act "Diva Celebrities" since 2016. Marilyn Monroe has been her favorite. She has performed

---

15 Rotten Tomatoes.com
16 Professional Beauty Newsletter, Joanna Sterkowicz, August 23, 2021
17 https://www.thebash.com/search/marilynmonroe-inpersonator-newjersey

on television and in large theaters "to the delight of audiences everywhere." She has performed in Europe, Asia, and "all over the USA," including "major Las Vegas and Atlantic City casinos." She graduated cum laude from the University of Portland. Past clients include the Giants, the Knicks, Bloomingdale's, Macy's, Zales Diamonds, Liz Claiborne, Calvin Klein, Turner Classic Movies, and the *Today* show.

She received a five-star review from Stacey F.: "Michelle performed as Marilyn Monroe for my husband's 65th birthday. She really made the party!! She was so fun to watch. She engaged everyone at the party in the fun, and my husband was so surprised. She was professional and gave out autographs to all the guests. I was very happy with the turn out, Michelle really made the party a success. Highly recommended."[18] And then there was Erica S. She has been performing in California since 2011, one of the top Marilyn Monroe impersonators in the world, known for her uncanny resemblance to the real Marilyn and her show-stopping performances.[19] An example of a review: "Erika was delightful and beyond expectations. Her rendition of Marilyn was spot-on and such great fun! She has a quick wit and so much talent. She was a huge hit with our crowd. She sings all of Marilyn's hit songs, including 'Diamonds are a Girl's Best Friend', 'I Wanna be Loved by You' and 'My Heart Belongs to Daddy.'"

Patriotic. She cut short her honeymoon on short notice to perform for the troops in Korea during the Korean War.[20] She did not go easy on herself, performing ten times over four days. She described her tour as "the best thing that ever happened to me."

She had her own library. Contrary to the stereotype of her as a "dumb blonde" who was just playing herself in her movies, she had a good intellect. She was a consistent reader and had organized her own library, which had over four hundred volumes. She was familiar with the work of many authors, including F. Scott Fitzgerald, John Steinbeck, and Tennessee Williams.

---

18   Ibid: VIEW PROFILE
19   Ibid: VIEW PROFILE
20   https://www.discoverwaelks.com/blog/united-states/top-10-shocking-facts-about-marilyn-monroe/.

She had *principles*, even having a contract canceled because she refused to be sexually exploited. Also, when her studio demanded that she break off her relationship with playwright Arthur Miller because he was being investigated by the House Un-American Activities Committee, she refused. Subsequently, the FBI opened a file on her. After her death, a sophisticated government-grade phone-tapping system that extended throughout her house was found.

Los Angeles Times[21]

Evidently, Marilyn just could not sleep, and in distress, she called her psychiatrist, Dr. Ralph Greenson, according to the police. He advised her to go for a ride. Subsequently, her maid, awakening at 3:00 a.m., noticed that Marilyn's bedroom light was still on. The maid addressed Marilyn but was met only with silence. Her door was locked. That's when she called Dr. Greenson, her psychiatrist, who came over and broke into her room. Marilyn was dead. There were several medicine bottles on her nightstand. One bottle was relatively new. It had contained forty Nembutal tablets but was now empty. (Nembutal is a barbiturate drug, one or two tablets of which could facilitate sleep but which, in much larger doses, can induce coma, respiratory depression, and death.)

In the article, it was noted "that medical authorities believed she had been in a depressed mood recently. It was described she was unkempt and in need of a manicure and pedicure, indicating listlessness and a lack of interest in maintaining her usual glamorous appearance." (Note: these symptoms are consistent with both addiction to barbiturates and, more particularly, entrenched, severe major depression in which suicidality could emerge as a real possibility.) And she had just been provided with a full bottle of Nembutal. In such circumstances, advice to "go for a ride" is medically and psychiatrically grossly inappropriate. And we lost her at merely thirty-six years old as a result. After her death, her psychiatrist commented, "I was under the impression she was going to take a ride to the beach or something like that."

---

21 From the Archives: Marilyn Monroe dies; Pills Blamed. Howard Hertel and Don Nef. The Los Angels Times. Aug. 6 1962 12 A.M. P.T.

The reporter was told that there had been approximately twelve to fifteen medicine bottles on her nightstand in addition to the emptied bottle of Nembutal.

Her body was transferred to the county morgue "where the nation's No. 1 glamour girl became coroner's case No. 81128, and her body was placed in Crypt 33. News of Miss Monroe's tragic death quickly circulated to much of the world. Even Moscow Radio made mention of it."[22]

Marilyn's career had been prospering. A proposal from Anita Loos, creator of *Gentlemen Prefer Blondes*, had just reached Marilyn. She could send her a script and music if she was interested. Another associate said that Marilyn had appeared in twenty-three movies since 1950, when she had a bit role in *The Asphalt Jungle*. He said that her movies had grossed over $200 million (at least $2 billion in 2022 dollars). "Does that sound like she was depressed about her career?" he queried. Miss Newcomb, Marilyn's press agent and close friend, reported that she had spent the Saturday before her death with her, and she had not noticed anything particularly disturbing about Marilyn's demeanor. After Marilyn's body was removed from her house, Miss Newcomb took possession of Marilyn's little beloved dog, Miff. All that was left behind were the dog's two stuffed toys, a tiger and a lamb.

The "Psychoanalyst"

After Marilyn's death, Joe DiMaggio expressed the sentiment that her Hollywood associates and contacts had treated her poorly and bore a responsibility for her death, but the real reasons lay in the realm of addictive illness and major depression.

In the year before her death, she was being "treated" by a "psychoanalyst." The definition in the *Britannica Dictionary*: "A doctor who helps people with mental and emotional problems by talking to them about their dreams, memories, etc. A doctor who practices psychoanalysis."[23] Psychoanalytic training is separate and different from the

22 Ibid., pg. 4-5.
23 Britannica Dictionary definition of Psychoanalyst.

training to become a specialist in medicine—for example, a surgeon, a dermatologist, or a psychiatrist. Many psychoanalysts first train to be psychiatrists, but psychoanalysts need not be physicians. PhDs can also apply to gain access to psychoanalytic training at a number of psychoanalytic institutes. It used to be highly prestigious to be admitted to a top psychoanalytic institute, particularly in the post-World War II period and into the 1970s or so.

Most psychiatrists who train in and practice psychoanalysis of necessity de-emphasize the medical side of psychiatry, which includes an emphasis on diagnosis, differential diagnosis, and varying levels of training in prescribing psychiatric drugs, but often not in clinical psychopharmacology, depending on the particular training institution. The latter, a new specialty, now contains a very large body of knowledge which cannot be "dabbled" in—what this author calls mere "pill prescribing," still the mode of practice for perhaps 80 percent of psychiatrists who have not invested the time and effort to master clinical psychopharmacology.

Unfortunately and fatally, Marilyn's treatment was conducted by a psychoanalyst in the year prior to her death. It's what wasn't done vis-à-vis her treatment that led to the tragic result. The undersigned must add that even if Marilyn's psychoanalyst had not been one—that is, was practicing "psychiatry"—a significant portion of psychiatrists also emphasize psychotherapy and are often "weak" on the medical-pharmacological side. And for those with serious so-called "mental" illness, that can be hazardous.

Marilyn had a history of substance abuse and brief hospital stays to be "detoxed." She had also been hospitalized for "depression."

In her final year, under the cloud of her barbiturate addiction, it was a matter of life and death that she have more treatment than just being detoxed. She needed to be encouraged, even cajoled, to accept admission into a longer-term recovery facility where, over several weeks, in the absence of the addicting substance, recovery methods are taught, building up the addict's resistance against using any addicting drugs upon discharge. (Otherwise, patients easily return to abuse.) Instead, the psychoanalyst responded to Marilyn's desperate situation by seeing her daily and even staying at her house overnight. It is very unclear what the doctor actually knew about addictive disease or how to effectively treat it, but his was not an adequate treatment response.

And then there was the clinical depression, and the synergy between it and addiction, as it was in Marilyn's case, can be deadly. If she had been in a recovery program, she should also have been assessed by a competent psychiatrist for the symptoms of major depression and potential suicidality. Both can be treated. That never occurred! And what a pity: her fame and wealth did not protect her.

The Funeral of Marilyn Monroe

Joe DiMaggio didn't hesitate to make the funeral arrangements. He flew right in. He decided none of Marilyn's Hollywood associates would be permitted to attend. He had a long-standing sentiment that they had treated her poorly and were indirectly responsible for her death.

The funeral was held at 1:00 p.m. on August 8, 1962, at the Westwood Village Memorial Chapel.[24] It was private. A Lutheran minister, A.J. Soldan, conducted the service. Readings were made from Psalms 46 and 139 and the Lord's Prayer. Tchaikovsky's Sixth Symphony and, at Marilyn's request, Judy Garland's "Over the Rainbow" were heard in the background.

As usual, Marilyn looked wonderful in her open bronze casket lined with champagne-colored satin. She wore her beloved green Pucci dress adorned with a green chiffon scarf. In Marilyn's hands were a "posy of pink teacup roses," a gift from DiMaggio, who sat in vigil the night before the funeral.

The eulogy was given by Lee Strasberg, her long-term acting coach but also close friend, like family:

---

24 http://www.marilynmonroe.ca/camera/about/facts/funeral.

Lee Strasberg
August 8, 1962, Westwood Memorial
Cemetery, Los Angeles, California

"Marilyn Monroe was a legend. In her own lifetime, she created a myth of what a poor girl from a deprived background could attain. For the entire world, she became a symbol of the eternal feminine."

"But I have no words to describe the myth and the legend, nor would she want us to do so. I did not know this Marilyn Monroe, nor did she."

"We gathered here today knew only Marilyn—a warm human being, impulsive and shy and lonely, sensitive and in fear of rejection yet ever avid for life and reaching out for fulfillment."

"I will not insult the privacy of your memory of her—a privacy she sought and treasured—by trying to describe her, whom you know, to you, who knew her. In our memories of her, she remains alive and not only a shadow on the screen or a glamorous personality."

"For us, Marilyn was a devoted and loyal friend, a colleague constantly reaching for perfection. We shared her pain and difficulties and some of her joys. She was a member of our family. It is difficult to accept the fact that her zest for life has been ended by this dreadful accident."

"Despite the heights and brilliance she had attained on the screen, she was planning for the future; she was looking forward to participating in the many exciting things which she planned. In her eyes and in mine, her career was just beginning. The dream of her talent, which she had nurtured as a child, was not a mirage."

"When she first came to me, I was amazed at the startling sensitivity which she possessed and which had remained fresh and undimmed, struggling to express itself despite the life to which she had been subjected. Others were as physically beautiful as she was, but there was obviously something more in her, something that people saw and recognized in her performances and with which they identified."

"She had a luminous quality—a combination of wistfulness, radiance, yearning—that set her apart and yet made everyone wish to be a part of it, to share in the childish naivete which was at once so shy and yet so vibrant."

"This quality was even more evident when she was on the stage. I am truly sorry that you and the public who loved her did not have the opportunity to see her as we did, in many of the roles that foreshadowed what she would have become. Without a doubt, she would have been one of the really great actresses of the stage."

"Now it is all at an end. I hope her death will stir sympathy and understanding for a sensitive artist and a woman who brought joy and pleasure to the world."

"I cannot say goodbye. Marilyn never liked goodbyes, but in the peculiar way she had of turning things around so that they faced reality—I will say *au revoir*."

"For the country to which she has gone, we must all someday visit."

My Story, by Marilyn Monroe

Marilyn Monroe with Ben Hecht. Taylor Trade Publishing, ©2007, Joshua Green. When Marilyn was merely two weeks old, her mother dropped her off at her first foster home. By the time she was sixteen, she had been in a succession of twelve and also an orphanage. The foster parents received $5 a week, perhaps $50-$100 dollars in current money (2022). Her mother made some effort to visit her in the foster homes, but it was difficult for her to be consistent due to symptoms of her "mental" illness and episodic hospitalizations.

On one occasion, her mother did manage to take Marilyn to her small bungalow. Marilyn was seven. There was a loud noise, and Marilyn saw that her mother had fallen down the stairs. She was "screaming and laughing." The police and an ambulance came. Marilyn was taken to an orphanage. Subsequently, over the years, she saw her mother only periodically. There was no father in evidence. But Marilyn believed she had a father. There was a picture in her mother's room. Her mother noticed Marilyn staring at it intently. "That's your father," she informed Marilyn.

"I felt so excited to have a father," Marilyn said. She knew "I belonged to him…He had a thin moustache like Clark Gable." She had a very warm feeling for the man in the picture. Her mother then told her he had died in a car accident. Marilyn refused to believe that. Her mother would not tell Marilyn the man's name. Nevertheless, Marilyn dreamed of the picture "a thousand times afterwards." Marilyn stated she learned more about him years later. He had lived in the same building as her mother; they fell in love, but when Marilyn "was getting born," he deserted them. Marilyn had no memory of him.

Some memories of those early years stand out. "Aunt Grace," a "make-believe relative," was a friend of her mother's who looked after Marilyn as best she could. She was kind but dirt-poor. At times, she brought Marilyn to her home for visits. On occasions, Grace used her last quarter to buy stale bread and some milk as their only sustenance. She and Marilyn would stand in line to buy "a sackful of bread at Holmes Bakery for twenty-five cents." Once, Marilyn looked up at her, and Grace said, "Don't worry, Norma Jeane; you're going to be a beautiful girl when you grow up."

She remembered her craving for attention, which manifested itself in church. As the organ was playing and the congregation was singing a hymn, she'd have an impulse to take off all her clothes so she would be standing "naked before God and everyone." She'd grit her teeth, sit on her hands, and vigorously implore God to stifle the impulse.

She remembered overhearing discussions about her family, that her mother, her grandfather, and her great uncle "had all been mental cases" and that she had a defective "heritage" and would end up the same way.

In all the foster homes, if the foster parents had their own children, she was used to being the "caboose," but one aspect of that stood out. Most of the families, being poor, bathed all the children in the same water. Marilyn, as usual, had the last bath and the dirtiest water.

She had only two similar dresses, both faded blue and white. When one was being cleaned, she wore the other. People would become annoyed because it appeared she never changed her dress.

She did have one favorite foster home. A great- grandmother, over a hundred years old, was the caretaker of the family's four children and also Marilyn. The great-grandmother was a great storyteller, riveting the children with "blood-curdling stories about Indian massacres, scalpings and burnings at the stake." Her last memory of that foster home was of one of the great-grandchildren accusing Marilyn of tearing her dress. Marilyn had not committed the act but was directly sent back to the orphanage.

An important source of emotional support was her own daydreaming, fantasies that she'd grow to become so beautiful "that people would turn to look at me when I pass." She'd dream she'd be wearing beautiful apparel in striking colors, scarlet, gold, green, and white, which would elicit admiration and praise from bystanders.

When she was nine, she was living with a family that had rented a room to a Mr. Kimmel, who appeared to be a respectable gentleman. One day, she was in the hall when his door opened. He asked her to come in, possibly to tell her of a task he wished her to do. But he took a key and locked the door when she was inside his room and stated, "Now you can't get out." She was afraid to scream. Mr. Kimmel was the "star boarder." She would not be believed and would be returned to the orphanage. She fought and kicked. Finally, he gave up and let her out. She hurried to tell her "aunt." "I want to tell you something," she stammered, "about Mr. Kimmel, he, he…" Her aunt did not allow her to finish the sentence, exclaiming, "Don't you dare say anything against Mr. Kimmel…he's a fine man. He's my star boarder."

Marilyn had a problem that perhaps many other young women would have liked to have had. At the age of twelve, she had the body and looks of a seventeen-year-old, and her secret wish had indeed come to pass: she was so beautiful.

She lived in a poor neighborhood. She had to walk to school, not having the requisite nickel for the bus. At school, she was ridiculed because of her shabby clothes, "my orphan's outfit." Once, she wore a borrowed sweater to school. It was too small for her. "In class, everybody stared at me as if I'd suddenly grown two heads." Then, at recess, "half a dozen boys crowded around me…they kept looking at my sweater as if it were a gold mine." She noted a marked rise in her popularity. "There were no sex thoughts on my mind…it was like a magic friend had appeared in my life." There was a side effect. The girls seemed more hostile, alarmed, perhaps, that Marilyn might poach their boyfriends. At the age of thirteen, "I had a real beau. I was able to fool him by keeping my mouth shut and walking a little fancy." And she had practiced her walk. "I had practiced walking languorously." And he took her to the beach, her first visit. "I stood and stared for a long time. It was like something in a dream, full of gold and lavender colors, blue and foaming white."

And because of the compulsive attention of all the boys, it occurred to her she must be a "siren." But she had no sexual thoughts at all. "I was as unsensual as a fossil." And she felt totally unprepared to be a siren. Her Aunt Grace made an unexpected suggestion: "You ought to get married." She suggested the young man next door, James Dougherty. Marilyn was living with her ninth set of foster parents, but they were moving out of state. "That would mean I'd have to go back to the orphanage."

She married Dougherty instead. It was like "being retired to a zoo." She further noted, "My husband and I hardly spoke to each other." The marriage was "pickled in silence." But she also was no longer a siren. The boys stayed away from Mrs. Dougherty.

It was the time of WWII. Jim, after joining the Merchant Marine, was shipped overseas in 1944. Marilyn got a job in a factory as a parachute inspector, for which she had to take a math class. "The men buzzed around me, just as the high school boys had done." She, however, was "completely faithful to my overseas husband." When Jim returned after the war, "he was a nice husband" except that "he wanted a baby. The thought of having a baby stood my hair on end." She was haunted; if she had a child, fate might color its life as it did for Norma Jeane, "still alone, still wishing she were dead."

As of the writing of *My Story*, she had developed a new perspective. "I feel different about having a child now. It's one of the things I dream of."

"This is the end of my story of Norma Jeane." She divorced Jim. She moved into a room by herself. "I was nineteen, and I wanted to find out who I was."

She had to look for a job. "The sort of instinct that leads a duck to water led me to photographers' studios." Financially, she was scrambling, sometimes not eating. "It didn't matter though. When you're young and healthy, a little hunger isn't important." But she was lonely. "I had no relatives to visit or chums to go to places with."

In a restaurant, she met an elderly man, a Mr. Bill Cox. They got to talking. He invited her for a visit to his home to meet his wife. She became friends with them. Bill Cox would tell her about the Spanish-American War, in which he served, and about Abraham Lincoln. She learned a great deal about the Spanish-American War, "its causes and all its battles." He went into detail about Abraham Lincoln "from his birth onward." But later, Bill told her he was moving to Texas. They corresponded, but then his wife sent her a letter; he had died. "The Hollywood streets seemed lonelier than ever without Bill Cox, San Juan and Abraham Lincoln."

"Sundays were the loneliest." When she was walking alone on one of those Sundays, she was near Union Station. Subsequently, on Sundays, she would go there to observe the people. They were largely poor. "You learned a lot looking at them. Good-looking men could have homely wives. Obviously burdened people with raggedy bundles and three or four sticky kids…had their faces light up like a Christmas tree when they saw each other." Really homely spouses, fat ones or old ones, "kiss each other as tenderly as if they were lovers in a movie."

She was taking acting lessons. She realized, "There must be thousands of girls sitting alone like me, dreaming of becoming a movie star…I'm dreaming the hardest." In the meantime, she took modeling jobs if available. And about the prospect of being a successful actress, she wrote, "Acting was something golden and beautiful…it enables you to step out of the dull world you know into worlds so bright, it makes your heart leap just to think of it."

But the Hollywood she knew at that point was the Hollywood of failure. "Nearly everybody I met suffered from malnutrition or suicide impulses." About the lady hopefuls, "We were the prettiest tribe of panhandlers that ever ran a town, and there were so many of us…homegrown sirens from every state of the Union." And they were plagued by wolves: "talent agents, press agents, contract men without contracts, and managers." The contracts they pushed "were usually a bedsheet." They were phony and failures, some vicious, "but they were as near to the movies I could get." There was Harry, a photographer, who enthusiastically informed her, "I know a real hot agent…he saw one of your stills and blew his top…he's crazy about you." Harry arranged a dinner for the three of them. He had prepped her that Mr. Laszlo had been the biggest agent in Budapest. The restaurant itself wasn't too promising, a cheap café. And Mr. Laszlo "was fat, unshaved, bald-headed, bleary-eyed, and his shirt collar was a little frayed," but he spoke with a fascinating accent. He was "ambitious" for her; she would not only be a big star but could "own [her] own movie studio and make only the finest movies…real art." He then made an offer, if she was willing to become a wife. The gentleman was elderly but a millionaire. He'd seen Marilyn's photographs. It would be a brief marriage; he was ailing. She would then inherit his estate; he had no relatives. Of his $2 million estate, Marilyn would keep half; he and Harry would split the rest.

Marilyn reflected, "Mr. Laszlo was one of the nicer scheme peddlers I met." All in all, there were over a dozen, some not as nice. One particular example was a Mr. Sylvester. He telephoned her and introduced himself as a talent scout for Samuel Goldwyn, the head of MGM Studios. He sounded authentic. He said she could fit well for a part in a planned movie. "It's not a big part, but very important." He picked her up and drove to the studio. However, it was 7:00 p.m., and there were not many people around. He led her to the office of a Mr. Dugan and gained entrance, reporting that he shared the office with Mr. Dugan. She noted the office was obviously for an important executive. Mr. Sylvester invited her to sit on the couch. He gave her a script and asked her to start reading. She used her most dramatic approach. As she kept reading, he requested she raise her skirt "a few inches," then to her knees, then to expose her thighs. She assumed that was reasonable as part of her audition. Next, he started "pawing me." She "socked him in the eye, jumped up, kicked him and banged my heel on his toes," and ran out.

Her automobile is what made it possible for her to visit the dozen studios and agents' offices to show her face. They were miles away from each other, but she could not afford to keep up the payments, and the car was repossessed pending a $50 payment. She "did everything possible to get the car back," even to the point of "calling up a few millionaires," but when she "started to dial one of their numbers, a hot, angry feeling filled me." But there was a stroke of luck. A photographer she knew called and made her aware of a job paying $50. "For fifty dollars, I am ready to jump off a roof," she exclaimed, but then she learned it would require her to pose nude. He assured her it will not be vulgar." Perhaps that was the famous calendar photograph. She got her car back!

She got a job as a bit player in a film, *Scudda Hoo! Scudda Hay!*, at 20th Century Fox. Her part was edited out. She knew she was "third rate...I could feel my lack of talent as if it were cheap clothing, but, my God, how I wanted to learn!" And she worked hard to improve her acting ability, spending her salary "on dramatic lessons, dancing lessons, and singing lessons." She studied books on acting. "I sneaked scripts off the set and sat up alone in my room reading them out loud in front of the mirror." A kindly assistant director on the set advised her to change her name from Norma Dougherty to something more glamorous. She liked the sound of Marilyn. Her mother's maiden name had been Monroe.

She met Mr. Schenck at a party. He was one of the prominent executives at 20th Century Fox. He invited her to his Beverly Hills mansion for dinner. "Then he fell into the habit" of inviting her two or three times a week. Rumors started that they were romantically involved, which was not the case. But she enjoyed his company. His friendship gave her "a great feeling of security."

But one morning, a casting official told her she was being dropped from the studio. "I couldn't talk. I was listening and couldn't move." She was told the head of the studio, Mr. Zanuck, had her cut out of all her pictures, deciding she wasn't "photogenic," that her looks are definitely against you." She believed she would learn to be an actress, "but how could I ever change my looks?" And she thought to herself, "Imagine how wrong my looks must be if even Mr. Schenck had to agree to fire me." She remained in bed "crying day after day...I got out of bed and looked in the mirror. Something horrible had happened. I wasn't attractive. I saw a coarse, crude-looking blonde." She was seeing what Mr. Zanuck must have seen. Her looks "were too big a handicap for a career in the movies." She felt "beaten" and ashamed. "I had tasted this feeling early, when a family would kick me out and send me back to the orphanage."

Surprisingly, Mr. Schenck invited her to dinner as usual and asked, "How are things going at the studio?" She was relieved that it was unlikely he played a role in firing her, and she told him bluntly, "I lost my job there last week." He encouraged her to "keep going." He told her of a possible job at X Studio. They hired her; their casting director was supportive, saying, "You ought to go a long way here. I'll watch out for a good part for you."

"I returned to my room…feeling alive again," Marilyn wrote. "And the daydreams started coming back—kind of on tiptoe." She later learned that Mr. Schenck had asked that head of another studio to do him a favor: hire Marilyn. She did a few bit parts as "background." She received a call from the casting director to come to his office at the studio. She was ushered into his office, but the casting director wasn't there. She anticipated that this could be her "big chance." She sat in a chair in the well-appointed office, "having dignity every minute." A door opened at the rear of the office. A man entered; she knew who he was, the head of X Studio, the equivalent of Mr. Zanuck at Fox. She told him she was waiting for Mr. A. "The hell with Mr. A," the great man exclaimed. She followed him to his office, which was "three time larger than Mr. A's." In his office, bedecked with Oscars and silver cups, he showed her a large photograph of a yacht, and he invited her on board for the evening. Marilyn said, "I'll be glad to join you and your wife on your yacht." He explained his wife would not be there. "What's the idea of standing there and staring at me?" he continued. "You're Joe Schenck's girl. He called me up to do him a favor and give you a job…is that a reason to get insulting?" Marilyn told him she was busy. He was standing and glaring at her. "I had never seen a man so angry." She left.

It was a low point. "The bottom of the ocean. When you're a failure in Hollywood, that's like starving to death outside a banquet hall with the smells of filet mignon driving you crazy." After the debacle with X Studio's head, she believed, "There was going to be no luck in my life…the dark star I was born under was going to get darker and darker. But there was a thing in me like a craziness that wouldn't let up. It kept speaking to me not in words, but in colors—scarlet and gold and shining white, green and blues." These were the colors that soothed Norma Jeane in the "dull world in which the orphanage slave existed."

One day in the office of a talent agency, a "very short man...with kind eyes" interviewed her, a Mr. Johnny Hyde. He informed her she reminded him of another talent he had discovered, Lana Turner. "You're better. You'll go further. You've got more."

She remarked, "Then why can't I get a job...just to make money to eat on?"

He assured her, "You're going to be a great movie star...you don't fit anything less...I can feel it...I see a hundred actresses a week." And a part opened up in John Huston's picture *The Asphalt Jungle*. Mr. Hyde brought her to Mr. Huston's office. "Mr. Huston was an exciting-looking man. He was tall, long-faced, and his hair was mussed." He gave her the script. Johnny asked her, "Do you think you can do it...you have to break up in it and cry and sob?" She studied the script. Next, she returned to Mr. Huston's office for a reading. "A pulse was pounding in my stomach." This was her first chance for a real acting part "with a great director."

After the reading, she was apprehensive, but "Mr. Huston caught my eye and grinned." He reassured her that she was in. "Go fix yourself up with the wardrobe department." She knew her part would not be cut out; "It was vital to the plot."

She described the role of a bit player. "In a movie, you act in little bits and pieces. You act two lines, and they say 'cut'...The minute you get going in your characterization, they cut." For the first time, however, she felt good to have a brief part in *The Asphalt Jungle* "because it was an adult script." Mr. Huston "was interested in the acting I did... Everything I did was important to him." Mr. Hyde was enthusiastic about her work. "This is it, honey. You're in. Everybody is crazy about your work." During the preview, she was very pleased with the movie, "It was a fine picture; I was thrilled by it." And she was pleased by the audience reaction to herself. "They laughed happily when I spoke.

They liked me very much." As for Johnny Hyde, "his heart was happy for me…when he put his arms around me and said he loved me, I knew it was true…I wished with all my heart I could love him back."

But then, a jolt: the studio, Metro, would not give her a contract. The studio liked her work, but they did not feel she was star material. Marilyn said, "Maybe they're right." Johnny emphatically said, "The studio is wrong…And so, was Zanuck…they'll eat their words someday." But she was reassured by having Johnny as her ally. He "swarmed all over the studios." But there was a clunker. "The love he hoped for wasn't in me. You might as well try to make yourself fly as to make yourself love."

And Johnny continued to swarm. He informed her, "We've landed a good one." It was a new Joseph Mankiewicz picture, *All About Eve*.

Wolves

One thing Marilyn had expertise in was the subject of wolves. But first, she had a rather idiosyncratic standard for all men. "I couldn't ever be attracted to a man with perfect teeth. A man with perfect teeth always alienated me." She speculated that "the kind of men I have known who had perfect teeth, they weren't so perfect elsewhere." She does find being made a pass at "is never entirely unpleasant, because men who make passes are usually bright and good-looking…There is variety among men. The nicest thing about wolves is that they seldom get angry or critical of you. This doesn't apply if you succumb to them. A wolf is inclined to get very angry if a woman makes the mistake of falling in love with them." One variety of wolf she thinks more highly of is "intellectual men who are full of ideas and information about life…It's always a delight to hear such men talking…then there are men who are total losses." They are the ones who indulge themselves "in plain, uninterrupted boasting, giving you an inside on what they like to eat and where they've been for the last five years…The real lover is the man who can thrill you by just touching your head or smiling into your eyes." And about women, "I have always had a talent for irritating women since I was fourteen…Wives have a tendency to go off like burglar alarms when they see their husbands talking to me." At parties, when a man speaks to her, "They think I'm plotting something…how to steal their gentlemen friends from under their noses." At some parties, men have avoided her, and "no one spoke to me for a whole evening…the men, frightened by their wives and sweeties, would give me a wide berth."

Johnny Hyde

She spent a lot of time with Johnny Hyde. "He took me everywhere." He wanted for them to get married. She was honest with him. "I don't love you, Johnny." She did all she could to lessen his hurt. She didn't date others during their relationship. She would do almost everything for him, but "he needed something I didn't have, love." He continued to propose marriage. He told her he was a millionaire, which she would inherit on his death. She would reassure him, "I'll not leave you. I'll never betray you. But I can't marry you." He was hospitalized. He was found to be seriously ill. He died. "His family wouldn't let me sit among them at the funeral." When she passed by his coffin, "I forgot myself. I threw myself on the coffin and sobbed. I wished I was dead with him." She had lost him, "the kindest man in the world."

One evening, she was eating dinner out with two friends, one a writer, the other a director. They were more or less talking to themselves about the artists Botticelli and Leonardo da Vinci, weighing their relative merits. One noticed that Marilyn seemed bored. "Let's talk about something closer to her than the Renaissance," the writer suggested. "How about sex?" They began discussing "Freud and Jung and a few other characters who seemed to me pretty mixed up." She thought to herself, "about two-thirds of the time, I hadn't the faintest idea of what people were talking about…There was no hiding it, I was terribly dumb." She knew nothing "about painting, music, books, history, geography…sports or politics." She enrolled at the University of Southern California to take a course in art. The teacher was a woman.

"I didn't think a woman could teach me anything." But Marilyn soon changed her mind. "She was one of the most exciting human beings I had ever met." Her discussion about the Renaissance was "ten times more important than the Studio's biggest epic. I drank in everything she said." She learned about Michelangelo, Raphael, and Tintoretto. "There was a new genius to hear about every day." She started buying books by, for example, "Freud and some of his disciples. I read them till I got dizzy." But her schedule was so full that she didn't have time. "I finally decided to postpone my intelligence." But when things quieted down, she promised herself she would "start learning—everything." She'd read voraciously. She would understand conversations and even "be able to contribute a few words."

And then, all her effort suddenly paid off. "Success came to me in a rush." The movie magazines "started printing my picture and giving me write-ups." But a hitch: "Just as I was beginning to go over with the public in a big way," she learned the nude calendar of her, which she had done anonymously, would be sold as a Marilyn Monroe novelty item. A friend, however, felt it would be a further boost for her. "The nude calendar is going to put you over with the biggest bang the town has heard in years." And he was correct. She was in great demand. She starred in two successful films, *Gentlemen Prefer Blondes* and *How to Marry a Millionaire*. And the studio, whose head had once told her she was not photogenic and would not succeed—well, his studio made a fortune with these two films in which Marilyn was the star! (So much for his good judgement!) And she got a raise to $1,200 a week(perhaps ten to twelve thousand in 2022 dollars). Finally, she could buy good-quality clothes. She now had "fame, money, and a future with all the publicity I could dream of. I even had a few friends." But "instead of being happy over all these fairy tale things…I grew depressed and finally desperate. My life suddenly seemed as wrong and unbearable to me as it had in the days of my early despairs."

She became her own self-critic of her lateness and other "bad social habits…Sometimes I know the truth of what I'm doing, it isn't

Marilyn Monroe but Norma Jean. I'm giving Norma Jean a treat."
She used to be the last to get a bath in the homes of her foster parents,
when the dirty, unpleasant bathwater had been used by six or eight
people. Now she could "bathe in water as clean and as transparent as a
pane of glass. And it seems Norma can't get enough of fresh bathwater
that smells of real perfume." And her lateness was also somewhat a
mystery. She became aware of "an impulse in me to be as late as possible...It makes something in me happy to be late...People are waiting
for me...I'm wanted. And I remember the years I was unwanted. All
the hundreds of times nobody wanted to see the little servant girl,
Norma Jeane, not even her mother." She received criticism for her
lateness, but for part of her, the Norma Jeane part, "the later I am, the
happier Norma Jeane grows."

"It was a difficult period, I felt tired all the time, worse, I felt
dull...What happened was that in working to make good, I had forgotten all about living." Her life was consumed with work. She had
neglected her need for other interests. Love was absent from her life,
only striving to succeed.

But then a friend at the studio mentioned that she knew of a gentleman Marilyn should get to know, Joe DiMaggio. Marilyn had heard
the name; "He's a football or baseball player." Her friend clarified, "He
is one of the greatest names in baseball." But Marilyn, at first, wasn't
interested. But she finally agreed to go to a party. DiMaggio would
also be there.

The host introduced them. "I was quite surprised; Mr. Joe
DiMaggio was unexpected." He wasn't "a loud or sporty fellow" but
quite conservatively dressed in an agreeable gray suit. They were seated
next to each other. She made conversation, remarking on his tie having
colorful blue polka dots. He responded, "Glad to meet you," but then
he "fell silent the whole of the rest of the evening." Other men at the
table "talked and threw their personalities around...Mr. DiMaggio
just sat there. Yet somehow, he was the most exciting man at the table." Then she noticed the other men were not paying attention to

her. "It was DiMaggio they were wooing…I had never met any man in Hollywood who got so much respect and attention at the dinner table." And she noticed she was no longer tired, even though she had been "dead tired" when she arrived at the party. She admitted to herself she was attracted to him. But she was perplexed by what exactly Mr. DiMaggio had done or did. But since he was so silent, she assumed there was no interest on his part. "The whole thing is a waste of time." Best is to go home "and forget him without delay." Then she excused herself, intending to leave. As she stood up, so did Mr. DiMaggio. "May I show you to the door?" He then accompanied her to her car. He said he had walked to the party but would appreciate a ride back to his hotel, which was close by, but then he suggested it was too early to turn in. Why not just go for a pleasant drive? Would she mind?

"Would I mind? My heart jumped." They drove for three hours. DiMaggio explained that he preferred to go out only once or twice with a woman. He had a friend, George Solitaire, who would then "run interference for me, and pried the girl loose."

Marilyn commented, "I'll try not to make him too much trouble when he starts prying me loose."

But Mr. DiMaggio replied, "I don't think I will have to use Mr. Solitaire's services this trip." He then complimented her; she was so pretty. She knew she was thought of as beautiful, "but this was the first time my heart jumped to hear it."

Publicity Episode

And then she had a publicity episode go awry. It was on behalf of the US Armed Forces. She wore a "regular afternoon dress…entirely decent. You could ride in a streetcar without disturbing the passengers." But one bright-minded "photographer" took a shot of her, pointing down from a balcony as she passed by. An army general saw the photograph and condemned it. It was too revealing of her bosom. She had not intended that. "Earl Wilson, who writes about bosoms" in the *New York Post*, interviewed her over the phone. He believed she had

THE INCREDIBLE SHRINKING BRAIN

deliberately leaned forward. She said it "was the photographer who leaned downward." Her final thought: "It was surprising a woman's bosom, slightly revealed, could become a matter of national concern. You would think that all the other women kept their bosoms in a vault." The photograph also drew crank letters from "Mr. and Mrs. Anonymous." Marilyn aptly named this episode the "bosom tempest."

Michael Chekhov

And she studied acting in depth from a master of the art, the famous Michael Chekhov. Under his tutelage, she reviewed a dozen plays. With Chekhov discussing "their characters and the many ways to play them," she realized acting was "an art that transformed you into somebody else." She loved it, was devoted to acting. But at one point, Michael stopped in midair and asked her an unexpected question. "Will you tell me truthfully, were you thinking of sex while we played the scene?" She denied she was at all. He commented while they rehearsed the scene, "I kept receiving sex vibrations from you." This upset Marilyn. It was her desire to be a serious actress. He said she was a young woman who gave off sex vibrations in spite of herself. "No matter what you are doing or thinking, the whole world has already responded to those vibrations," and that explains the stereotyped roles the studio wants her to play, "and your studio bosses are only interested in your sex vibrations, they care nothing about you as an actress. You can make them a fortune by merely vibrating in front of the camera." She didn't even have to act. Marilyn reacted to his summation by saying, "I want to be an artist, not an erotic freak. I don't want to be sold to the public as a celluloid aphrodisiac…that makes a fortune for the studio sex peddlers."

For her next movie, the notorious Mr. Zanuck would not even give her the script to review ahead of time. When she specifically asked for the script, she was informed that "Mr. Zanuck didn't consider it necessary for me to see the script in advance." She learned of the title, *The Girl in Pink Tights*. The title was a concern, with the studio evidently planning to spike her "vibrations" by having her wear them as a major publicity effort. She demanded the script and was again denied it, but finally they sent it to her. "It was silly…below dullness." She was to play "this dreary cliché-sprouting bore in pink tights… the cheapest character" she had read in any script.

Furthermore, "when I think of Joe and my friends seeing me on the screen as this rear-wiggling schoolteacher doing bumps and grinds…I blush to my toes." She refused the part. She was not about to be a "freak" performer.

Joe

But she and Joe were increasingly committed to each other. Finally, it seemed to make sense to get married. He suggested that she accompany him to Japan, where he had business, and then they would make a honeymoon of the rest of the time. If the studio situation was uncertain, up in the air, she was certain of one thing: "What Joe is to me is a man whose looks and character I love with all my heart."

And if there was one thing Joe was certain about, it was that he hated publicity and had avoided it as much as possible during his career. But publicity stuck to Marilyn like a parasite. They found out it was big news in the media that she had a falling-out with the studio. She was upset. "Seeing your name in front page headlines as if you were some kind of major accident or a gun battle is always startling… you keep thinking, the whole country's reading about me, maybe the world."

She was hoping to see Japan, as she had no further publicity demands from the studio. But she had to reckon with the United States Army. A General Christenberry was on their flight to Japan, and he approached them before they landed in Tokyo and inquired, "How would you like to entertain the soldiers in Korea?" Joe said he would like to, but his schedule would not permit it. The general politely said he was inquiring of Ms. Monroe. So, she was flown to Korea while Joe remained in Tokyo. Her first stop was at a hospital to perform for wounded soldiers. She left very pleased to have entertained them, and they in turn were enthusiastic. But the officer in charge of her tour had a complaint about one of her songs, "Do It Again," saying that it was too suggestive for young men. She explained it was a Gershwin song, but the officer let her keep it in her act only when she suggested changing the lyric to "Kiss me again" and avoided "putting any suggestive meaning into it." And she never did get a chance to see the real Korea, being flown by a helicopter from one base to the next. She remembered, in particular, her performance at the 45th Division. An officer had come backstage. "You'll have to go on ahead of schedule…I don't think we can hold them off any longer. They're throwing rocks on the stage." And the roar she heard was her name being screamed. She performed a cute dance. "I knew they would like it."

"This is where Marilyn's manuscript ended when she gave it to me," wrote Milton H. Greene.

Carrie Fisher—Her Death

Headline, *Los Angeles Times*,[25] "Carrie Fisher's autopsy reveals cocktail of drugs, including cocaine opiates and Ecstasy." She was returning from London to Los Angeles when she reportedly stopped breathing, according to another passenger, as the plane was about to land. The Los Angeles Fire Department was at the gate when the plane landed, responding to a cardiac arrest on board. She was immediately taken to a hospital. She hung on for four days and was thought to be stable but then died on December 27, 2016. She was sixty years old.

Reportedly, she had been diagnosed with bipolar disorder decades earlier. She also obviously had an addiction. She was a creative, intelligent woman, but had any psychiatrist ever told her the morbid risks she was taking using powerful street drugs, dangerous in their own right but poisonous to the brain of a person with a confirmed diagnosis of a bipolar disorder? Had any psychiatrist ever told her there are evidence-based medications that stabilize bipolar disorder? There is no mention that she was taking appropriate medications. Such medications, which can also be measured in the blood, could include what are called mood-stabilizers. There are a number of them that can be used individually or in combinations. They are evidence-based (scientifically demonstrated) to reduce the number and severity of depressive, hypomanic, and manic episodes. Lithium, the oldest medication, also has anti-suicidal properties.

25 http://www.latimes.com/locafl/lanow/la-me-in-carrie-fisher-autopsy-report-20170619-story.html.

She was the daughter of two celebrities, Eddie Fisher, one of the most popular singers during the 1950s, who sold millions of records, and Debbie Reynolds, an actress, singer, dancer, and businesswoman whose career spanned seventy years.

It was not long after her birth that Elizabeth Rosemond Taylor entered her life, although initially indirectly. Born in London on February 27, 1932, Taylor was one of film's most celebrated actresses, exceptionally beautiful but also a talented actress, playing complex characters in her movies. But she wasn't immune to tragedy. Her husband, film producer Mike Todd, died in a plane crash. Debbie, who had met Elizabeth, wanted Eddie to drop by to offer condolences. Debbie, later reflecting back on her life for an HBO special, *Wishful Drinking*, commented, "Eddie rushed to Taylor's side, gradually moving to her front."[26]

Debbie's son, Todd, Carrie's brother, described the consequences as "one of Hollywood's biggest notorious scandals." When Eddie left, Carrie was too small to grasp the situation. "The affair blazed on, and Eddie left Debbie alone to bring up their two children." This did not help Eddie's reputation; he was referred to in some quarters as a "philandering, opportunistic loser." Eddie became Elizabeth's fourth husband.

Carrie accepted Eddie's and Elizabeth's marriage. "I never felt bitter about Elizabeth…A man doesn't leave a woman for another woman unless he wants to go." By 1963, four years after they got married, Elizabeth met Richard Burton on the set of Cleopatra. Their affair "would ultimately outlast all of her seven marriages" (including the one with Fisher). Carrie's life and career were influenced by her mother, Debbie Reynolds. Their relationship underwent cycles but ended on an endearing note. Carrie's birth in 1956 was a news item because of her mother's fame. A photograph taken when she was six "showed her enraptured by Reynolds performing in Las Vegas."[27] But as Carrie grew older, she began to resent her mother's fame. Her mother

26 https://www.mirror-co.uk/3am/celebrity-elizabe4th-taylor's red-hat-mirror.
27 https://www.biography.com/news/carrie-fisher-debbie-reynolds-relationship.

commented on that period. "She wanted a mother who baked and did embroidery. I was in show business and didn't do that." Carrie later explained, "I had to share her, and I didn't like that. When we went out, people sort of walked over me to get to her. And I didn't like it." When Carrie was thirteen, however, she joined her mother's performances at night clubs in Las Vegas. In 1975, she landed a part in the movie *Shampoo*, playing a love interest of Warren Beatty. Deborah wanted to be certain Beatty did not duplicate that in real life, telling Beatty, "If you touch her, I will take out a hit on you."

But the mother-daughter relationship hit a very rough patch in Carrie's twenties. They were estranged for nearly ten years. "We had a fairly volatile relationship earlier on in my twenties," Carrie told Oprah Winfrey in 2011. "I didn't want to be around her. I did not want to be Debbie Reynolds's daughter." Subsequently, Carrie reflected that her mother was "a very powerful person," and she wanted to develop her own identity. "I had to forge some kind of character out of nothing."

Deborah told Oprah, "My lowest point in Carrie's and my relationship was probably when we discovered she was ill, that she had this mental health problem and that it's going to be with her forever…How is she going to get along in life?…All I could do is love her, and I always shall." Carrie had been diagnosed with bipolar disorder in her twenties (henceforth to be categorized by organized psychiatry as "mentally ill," or, if you will, "a mental case"). And unfortunately, clouding that "mental" illness was Carrie's early use of street drugs, LSD, cocaine, heroin, and painkillers. When she was twenty-eight, she entered a rehabilitation facility for the first time. Evidently, there were subsequent rehabs (repeat rehab admissions are not unusual for severe addiction), but in Carrie's case, bipolar disorder and active addiction eventually killed her. The real question is, did she have to die? Her mother made it to eighty-four, then died of grief. There was possibly a lopped-off quarter century of Carrie's life span.

But in spite of these torments, by dint of will, intelligence, and extraordinary creativity, Carrie did manage to push her career along.

She wrote a novel in 1987, *Postcards From the Edge*, which, in 1990, was adapted into a feature film starring Meryl Streep. In 2001, Carrie wrote a television movie from her book, starring her mother. Debbie did not take offense to the content, stating that "it took thirty years for Carrie to be really happy with me." Deborah bought a house right next to Carrie's. They remained neighbors until their deaths. They had developed a close and mutually admiring relationship.

Of course, Carrie's most memorable part in media was as Princess Leia in the *Star Wars* series.

Carrie Fisher Opens Up About *Star Wars*[28]
Author Interviews

In 2016, *Fresh Air* host Terry Gross interviewed Fisher, who played Princess Leia opposite Harrison Ford, as Han Solo, in the first *Star Wars* episode. She had just written a book, *The Princess Diarist*, about the shooting of the episode, during which she had a secret affair with Harrison Ford. She had placed the diary that she had incorporated into the book in a box and then forgotten about it. She subsequently located it again. Gross asked her what her reaction was upon rereading it. It made her realize how insecure she had been. She didn't really know who she was. Gross pointed out that she had been the only girl in an "all-boy fantasy." She asked her when she realized she had been the object of boys' sexual fantasies. Fisher replied that it had not occurred to her until eight years later, "when some guy said to me, 'I thought about you every day from when I was twelve to twenty-two.'"

She asked him, "Every day?"

He replied, "Four times a day." Gross noted that *The Princess Diarist* had a lot of material about her affair with Harrison Ford. Had he read it before it was published? Fisher had sent it to him, but he never responded. She commented about him that he was a private person, non-disclosing, not talking a lot. The relationship "was going nowhere. It was sort of half a conversation." Gross commented that

---

28   The Gold Bikini And Her On-Set Affair, NPR, November 28, 2016.

she had described Ford as being "like a fantasy for you, but the fantasy didn't always work out." She asked her to read a passage in the diary about their relationship.

"We have no feeling for one another," Fisher read. "We lie buried together during the night and haunt each other by day, acting out something that we don't feel and seeing through something that doesn't deserve any focus. I have never done anything quite like this. I sit patiently awaiting the consequences. I talk, walk, eat, sleep, patiently awaiting the consequences. How can a thing that doesn't seem to be happening come to an end? George says that if you look at the person that someone chooses to have a relationship with, you'll see what they think of themselves. So, Harrison is what I think of myself. It's hardly a relationship, but nevertheless, he is a choice. I examined all the options and chose the most likely to leave no emotional investments. Never love for me, only obsession. Someone has to stand still for you to love them. My choices are always on the run."

Gross thanked her for reading the passage and observed that she chose someone who was "not invested in you." And she noted "you're having an affair, so how did the affair affect the chemistry on the screen?" Fisher said it seemed to facilitate their acting: "There was chemistry there, you can see it." Gross noted that their characters even had a child. Yes, she and Harrison "had Hitler as a child, who did not resemble either one—for one thing he was 6 foot 5 inches tall." Gross observed the book seemed to indicate she had "a kind of love-hate relationship with your identity as Princess Leia." Carrie corrected her, saying she really liked the character, how she treated people, her honesty, her competence. But there was one distracting downside, the hair conundrum. Gross asked her what she saw when she looked in the mirror, "a giant, fat face like a sanddab with features." And she replied, "the horrible hair, I just looked like—I don't know, like this really fat-faced, cute-in-a-not-good-way girl." Gross asked who cooked up the idea of putting buns on both sides of her head. They were trying out several different hairstyles. "Somehow, they chose that one. And to put more hair on either side of a round face is going to make it even wider. So that was my problem with that."

Gross, since they were discussing appearance, remarked, "In *Return of the Jedi*, you were wearing this incredibly revealing metal bikini… in which you looked rail-thin" while sitting on the lap of "this giant, slimy, slug-like creature and crime boss…who is toying with you. He's kind of, like, petting you and licking his lips…" Carrie commented that he didn't have lips. Gross continued, "There's so, like, something sexual about it." It was a movie for kids, yet with the deeper S&M imagery of the scenes, was it appropriate?" That's how they rehearsed it. Jabba first talks to Harrison and Mark, who are then led away. "Sure, they'll be digested, but I have to stay with the slug with the big tongue." Gross commented, "And nearly naked." Carrie said she thought they were kidding about wearing the skimpy metal bikini. It wasn't her choice. They insisted. But there was a redeeming aspect: she got to kill the slug, "which was so enjoyable. I sawed his neck off with the chain that I killed him with…I couldn't wait to kill him."

The conversation turned to her mother, Debbie Reynolds's, ill health. She had two strokes. Gross asked, "Did she come close to dying?" Carrie described her mother's difficult year; she also had an infection in her spine, and she got pneumonia. It did seem she might die. At one point, she could only say two words, but somehow, "She came back. She's fully back." Carrie further commented that her mother hates nurses. "They were telling her what to do, and no one tells my mother what to do." She would yell at the nurses. She told her, "Mom, not cool." Of course, the year was traumatic for both of them. Carrie could not concentrate sufficiently to continue writing. She reflected about her mother, "There are very few women from her generation who worked like that, who just kept a career going all her life and raised children and had horrible relationships and lost all her money and got it back again. I mean, she's had an amazing life, and she's someone to admire."

Gross asked her opinion about the movie *Singing in the Rain*, one of the great musicals of all time, in which her mother starred. "I always liked it. It's brilliant." She commented that the musical and *Star Wars* had a commonality, each having three people acting in them, two men and a woman, and each was rated by the AFI as one of the ten top films.

The topic turned to Carrie's relationships with men. Gross commented, "You write that you felt doomed to have bad relationships with men." That was her entire experience. Her father, Eddie Fisher, walked out on them when she was a toddler. Her mother had a disastrous second marriage, with her second husband swindling her out of all her money and Reynolds ending up having to pay off his substantial debts with her future earnings. That gem of a husband, whose name was Harry Karl, had people over to their home he had described as a barber and manicurists. It turned out the "barber" was a pimp, "so he was having a lot of hookers at the house."

Carrie commented, "Well, yes, I hated him. And then we stayed living with him, until finally, even though it took a really long time for her to leave him," both she and her mother slipped out, going to New York. "He didn't know she [her mother] was getting a divorce…It was very complicated, not something you want to do again."

Gross then asked about her relationship with her father, Eddie Fisher, since he left when she was going on two. They never had a "father-daughter relationship." It was only when he was elderly that "I had a mother-son relationship with him," taking care of him when he was ill. Evidently, Eddie also abused drugs. "He took drugs all his life and shot speed and so forth." In his more frail years, "He smoked pot all the time…so we called him 'Puff Daddy.'" Of course, she had always longed for a relationship with him, so she took it on any terms she could, becoming his nurse.

Changing the topic, Gross asked about her bipolar illness. "And you know, I've read you had ECT—electro-convulsive therapy—shock treatment." She had heard that "it would just erase people's memories."

Carrie informed Gross, "There is no convulsion anymore…it's actually very effective, but it has such stigma. It's unbelievable." Gross asked her if it helped her. "It did, absolutely. You know, it was the big thing to have done, so I would have had to be in a lot of trouble to consider it…It was very effective." She had been very depressed, and medication wasn't working, "so I utilized it. But it was hard to decide to do it because of all the stigma attached to it."

She asked her, since she had been so open about the personal details of her life, if there had been untoward consequences. No, it was her way of promoting self-understanding, and she also found that others positively responded to her. Also, she learned her private issues weren't unique.

Then the pièce de resistance. Gross inquired about her dog, Gary, who was with her in the studio. Gross commented, "You get to take him everywhere…I didn't know they usually let dogs in the NPR studio." she inquired if Gary was an official therapy dog.

"He is," but his best trait was that "he's very soothing to have around. He's licking my hand right now. He's just very nice to have around."

Gross exclaimed, "Oh my God, I hear him licking your hand… that is such a loud lick."

She noted, "Well, he has a very big tongue…a very, very long tongue." He goes with her on planes. He'll sit on the seat, and she'll sit on the floor. Gross inquired how she met him. She got him in New York, in the Village, "at a very tragic pet store. He looked like he was from a puppy mill, everything is sort of wrong with him." Gross asked what about Gary attracted her. "The tongue…it just got longer and longer and never went into his mouth." Evidently, Gary was still licking her.

"I can't believe I still hear him licking you."

"He's the most well-behaved dog I've ever had…he can give you a high five…he sits like Winston Churchill."

Gross then changed the subject, asking her about Comic–Con conventions—when others imitate Princess Leia, what are their costumes and hairdos like? Carrie replied, "My favorite is seeing men in the metal bikini, often bulky men."

Gross replied, "That's hilarious."

Carrie added, "Not only is Princess Leia fatter, she's a guy." Gross thanked her for the interview. She replied, "Thanks for talking to me." He also gave his regards to Gary. Carrie said, "I'll lick him for you."

This accomplished, intelligent woman so mismanaged her bipolar illness after decades of having it that it makes one think there were catastrophic lapses in the treatment of it, and also of her addiction, on the part of her psychiatrists. She should not have died. One can regard the use of street drugs and the absence of an appropriate treatment regimen as causing indirect suicide, in which her psychiatrists shared responsibility.

What she required in order to stabilize her disorders and save her life would have been a psychiatrist, years before she died, who made a serious "intervention" in the presence of the patient *and* her significant others, and an extended session could have been arranged in which it was explained in detail: the therapeutic path she must take, with detoxification to start, but then a sustained period of addiction rehabilitation, possibly three months. Once she was completely detoxed, then an expert psychopharmacologist could have planned an appropriate pharmacological mood-stabilizing regimen for the bipolar illness. But instead, her "treatment" appears to have been insufficient, inconsistent, and inadequate. The most appropriate summary: death by psychiatric incompetence.

Anthony Martin Bourdain
(June 25, 1956-June 28, 2018)

Bourdain and his collaborator, Eric Ripert, were on location in Kaysersberg-Vignoble, France, filming an episode of Bourdain's very successful TV travel-documentary *Parts Unknown*. Mr. Ripert had been expecting Bourdain to join him for breakfast, their usual routine, but grew concerned when Bourdain failed to show up. Mr. Ripert decided to go up to Mr. Bourdain's hotel room. "America's most beloved travel guide was already gone."[29] He had hung himself using the belt of his hotel bathrobe. He was sixty-one. And so ended the life of one who *Smithsonian Magazine* had declared "was the original rock star of the culinary world." His successful suicide was a shocking surprise to many. His mother, Gladys Bourdain, was quoted in *The New York Times*: "He is absolutely the last person in the world I would have ever dreamed of would do something like this."

He was born in New York City to a Jewish mother and a father of French descent whose grandfather had come to the United Sates at the turn of the twentieth century. Both parents had responsible jobs. Gladys was a staff editor of *The New York Times*, his father an executive at Columbia Records. Bourdain described his childhood by saying, "I did not want for love or attention. My parents loved me. Neither of them drank to excess. Nobody beat me. God was

---

29   Anthony Bourdain, Wikipedia.

never mentioned, so I was annoyed by neither church nor any notion of sin or damnation."

As a youth, he was not the stay-at-home type. He had been an active boy scout. When older, he earned a blue belt in Brazilian jiu-jitsu, and later a gold. He had sunk into a period of drug abuse in his twenties—heroin, cocaine and LSD—but was able to stop them on his own before undergoing a noticeable deterioration in his health or functioning. He did continue to use marijuana and alcohol.

His father would travel to France, and when Anthony was old enough, he took him along. They were on a fisherman's boat when Anthony was offered a freshly caught oyster. The taste of it, to him, was a defining experience. He knew he must be involved with food more than three meals a day. He was accepted at Vassar College but enjoyed working at the seafood restaurants in Provincetown, Massachusetts, and dropped out of college after two years. In 1978, he graduated from the Culinary Institute of America. He went on to run several restaurant kitchens in Manhattan, including The Supper Club, One Fifth Avenue, and Sullivan's. In 1998, he was appointed as the executive chef at Brasserie Les Halles. It served classic French dishes such as escargot, foie gras, and steak tartare.

Writing Career

He started submitting unsolicited articles to various magazines and publishers in the mid-1980s. His first published article was about a prominent chef going downtown to purchase heroin. In 1999, his article in the *New Yorker* magazine, "Don't Eat Before Reading This," attracted attention. Soon afterward, he wrote an expanded version for his book *Kitchen Confidential: Adventures in the Culinary Underbelly*. It became a bestseller in 2000. He soon became a widely published author, even deviating from culinary topics to write two mysteries, *Bone in the Throat* and *Gone Bamboo*. Even though he paid for his own book tours, they did not catch on. But in his area of expertise, his books were popular: *A Cook's Tour*, *Nasty Bits* (a collection of thirty-seven exotic, provocative, and humorous anecdotes and essays), *Typhoid Mary: An Urban Historical*, and *No Reservations: Around the World on an Empty Stomach*. He had numerous articles published in magazines such as *The New York Times Magazine*, *The Los Angeles Times Magazine*, *The Observer*, *Gourmet*, *Maxim*, *Esquire*, *Scotland Sunday*, *The Face*, *Food Arts*, *Limb by Limb*, *Black Book*, *The Independent*, *Best Life*, *The Financial Times*, and *Town and Country*.[30]

He hosted his first television show, *A Cook's Tour*, in 2002. It ran for thirty-five episodes. In 2005, he introduced a new series, *Anthony Bourdain: No Reservations*. An episode was being filmed in Beirut, Lebanon, when war broke out between Israel and Lebanon. He and his staff were taken prisoner by Hezbollah and confined to a hotel. After several days, they were freed by United States Marines. Before he contracted with CNN in 2013 for his series *Parts Unknown*, he did many travel pieces for the Travel Channel. In 2015, he was in a scene in the feature film *The Big Short* in which he prepared an elaborate fish stew that was compared to a complex financial product, a collateralized debt obligation, which is assembled out of various loans, making up a pool of them to be sold as one product to investors.

Of course, he was best known for *Parts Unknown*, which ran on CNN from 2013 until his death in 2018. Always charming, he escorted his audience to every continent except Antarctica to learn of numerous, often exotic local cuisines and dishes while engaging with the most notable chefs. His death left a hole in that television slot, although they play reruns.

His personal life was not nearly as smooth as his professional life. He acknowledged he had abused heroin, cocaine, and LSD in the 1980s at a local restaurant with his friends. In the 1970s, while in high school, he had a crush on one Nancy Putkowski, and that's how he enrolled at Vassar—to follow her, as Vassar had just started admitting men. In April 2007, he married Ottavia Busia, with whom he had his daughter, Ariane. They separated in 2016. He met the Italian actress

---

30

Asia Argento[31] in 2016 while filming an episode of *Parts Unknown* in Rome, Italy. She seems to have been an unusual individual, having told the Italian media she was raped by the notorious Harvey Weinstein while attending the Cannes Film Festival when she was twenty-one. Reportedly, some Italian media outlets criticized her regarding this accusation, whereupon she left Italy to reside in Germany "to escape a culture of victim-blaming," as she put it.

Bourdain seemed particularly happy when he spent time with Argento. "He was clearly overjoyed to begin a new romance with her." The relationship was a positive development, but he "continued to struggle with his mental health." He often brought up death, wondering out loud how he would die and how he would kill himself if he decided to end his own life. In one of his last interviews, he said he was going to "die in the saddle." Bourdain is described, despite his enviable career, as being haunted by a darkness that he couldn't seem to shake. His friend, Eric Ripert, discovered Bourdain hanging in his hotel room. He expressed his sincere sentiment:

"Anthony was a dear friend. He was an exceptional human being, so inspiring and generous. One of the great storytellers of our time who connected with so many. I wish him peace. My love and prayers are with his family, friends, and loved ones."

This author's perspective is that he died of a disease that was not framed as a disease, instead being referred to as a "struggle with mental health" or being "haunted by a darkness." This is because psychiatry remains wedded to its scientifically inaccurate and stigmatizing classification that Bourdain was "mentally ill;" in other words, he was a "mental case," and of course, Margaritoff is under psychiatry's influence, as is the entire culture. It is possible Bourdain could not countenance labelling himself as a "mental case." He never received competent diagnosis or treatment for major depression. He reaped the whirlwind of a stigmatizing classification.

---

31 "The Story of Anthony Bourdain's Death and the Downward Spiral That Preceded It," Marco Margaritoff, 7/8/21. All that's interesting.com/Anthony-bourdain-death.

Dr. Stanton Peele, PhD, supplies a reasonable speculation about Bourdain's suicide.[32] "In spite of his past history of drug abuse, his toxicology screen after the suicide was negative. His involvement with Asia Argento since 2017 was of special significance. His love for her was evident among the people who worked with him. He would rave about Rome, where his girlfriend lived." His photographer, David Holloway, was quoted: "He would say it's an amazing city to fall in love in." Some of his friends, however, were unsettled by the intensity of his feelings for her: "Like a teenage boy, he was absolutely lovestruck. He would have done anything for her." Their love seemed to flourish, however. "Anthony Bourdain and Asia Argento seemed as tight as ever just last week…but it appears something changed in the last few days." As Bourdain was shooting in France, "Asia was back in Rome, strolling around with a French reporter…there were photos of them holding hands and hugging." Dr. Peele speculates that when Bourdain saw these paparazzi photographs in the paper, he reacted strongly, intensely. It's as if his love life with Argento had become all-consuming, even to the point of emotionally forgetting his eleven-year-old daughter. He was in a state of being submerged in feelings of loss, abandonment, and humiliation so painful that he could see no way out. That was the impact of seeing the photos of Argento "being cozy in various parts of the city, dancing together at a bar, holding hands, nuzzled up close together with this other man." Dr. Peele continued, "Combine that with his depressive loneliness, heartbreak, and the humiliation of this tough man wearing his heart on his sleeve for all the world to see how giddy he was to be with this woman, and I can see it is one thing more than he could bear at that moment for this impulsive act."

His suicide was triggered by the loss (in his mind) of the relationship, a feature of a condition Dr. Peele called "love addiction." And this was certainly a relevant aspect, but it was in the context of a major depressive illness, which is a real disease, a potentially fatal brain disease, which, in Bourdain's case, was fatal. It is more than a "mental

---

32   What killed Anthony Bourdain? Stanton Peele, PhD, https;//psychologytoday.com.

health" problem or an addiction. It is doubtful that it was competently diagnosed, let alone appropriately treated. In other words, a biophysiological, pathological process was occurring in his brain, hyperapoptosis, which was never thought of, never considered, and never treated. Bourdain was a victim of anachronistic psychiatry. He never knew what hit him. He died totally ignorant of what drove him to commit suicide.

Psychiatry frames major depressive illness as a "mental problem." It is unlikely Mr. Bourdain, a dynamic, creative, successful man, could have ever accepted being diagnosed as "mentally ill." But instead, if psychiatry reframed it as a neurological-like brain disease? (Not a "mental" problem?)

There was no competent provider to take his history and explain major depression and the effective treatment. Two years before his death, he had been in Buenos Aires, Argentina, shooting an episode of *Parts Unknown*. In the context of that episode, he disclosed that he had told a therapist, "Something as small as eating a bad hamburger could send me into a spiral of depression that can last for days." This was an important item of clinical information but led nowhere.

How would Sigmund Freud have handled Mr. Bourdain's case if he were practicing today? A fantasy speculation:

Freud was a neurologist, both an astute clinician and a successful researcher. He left no stone unturned in seeking to uncover and discover the biological etiologies for "mental" symptoms. In other words, it was to neurological explanations he turned first. But on a practical basis, he learned quickly that technological deficiencies stymied all his efforts. He then made a startling turn in direction, his genius manifesting in a brilliant, novel theory in his era.

But what if instead he were practicing in the modern era? Certainly, he'd be thrilled at the burgeoning of neuroscience, and given his instincts to hone in on the most critical neuroscientific information, he would realize that apoptosis gone awry was a fundamental cause of severe psychiatric illnesses, and he would make a beeline to the relevant research institute to dig in on that topic. In his clinical practice, he'd insist on careful, accurate diagnosis and differential diagnosis. He'd be a master of the medical treatments—that is, sophisticated clinical psychopharmacology. It is doubtful he would bother with "psychoanalysis," leaving that to the disciplines of psychology and social work. He started out as a physician in his time, but in our era, he would remain a physician throughout his career, a neurologically oriented psychiatrist—that is, a clinical psychopharmacologist.

If only Mr. Bourdain had encountered such a physician, an enlightened psychiatrist, in a situation in which going to a psychiatrist paralleled going to a neurologist for neurological symptoms. The neurologist is a student of the brain and its pathophysiological dysregulations. First and foremost, he makes a careful diagnosis. He uses advanced pharmacological treatments to relieve painful symptoms and forestall injury to brain tissue. In contrast, the majority of psychiatrists suffer from "dual identity pathology." (Which are they, therapists or physicians?) Unlike neurologists, they are unfamiliar with the details of brain dysregulations. Most have never heard of hyperapoptosis. They "pill-prescribe" but have not mastered the details of the medical specialty, clinical psychopharmacology. Psychiatry as a specialty suffers from a "dual identity pathological disorder" not to be found in their diagnostic manual, the DSM. The "therapist" identity interferes with the medical identity, which is undeveloped in comparison to all the true medical specialties like neurology, internal medicine, or endocrinology. They fail to recognize the physical damage in the brain occurring in the major disorders they're responsible for—schizophrenia, bipolar disorder, and severe major depression.

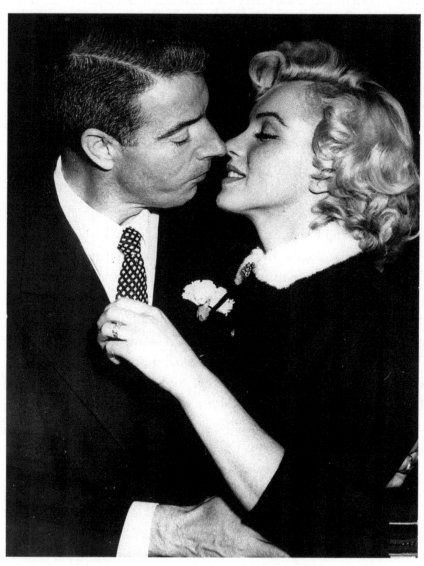

Monroe DiMaggio Wedding

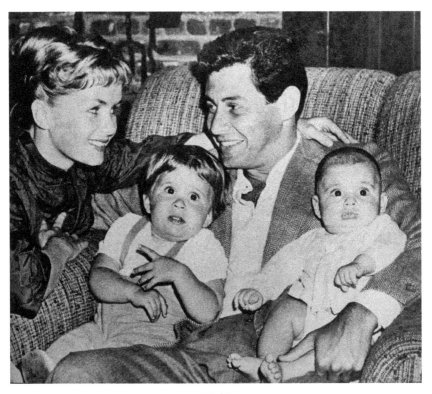

1958

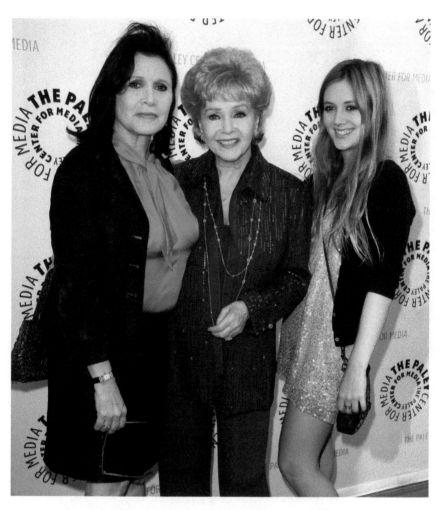

Carrie Fisher (L), Debbie Reynolds, and Billie Lourd

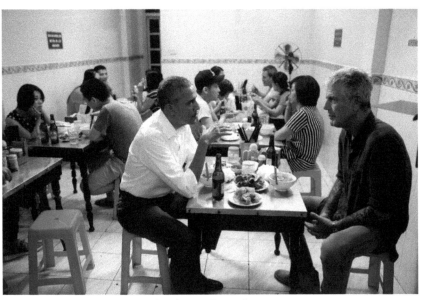

Anthony Bourdain

Potential Blood Biomarkers for Suicidality

Who would have known genes (which are physical entities) would play such an influential role in suicidality? But this is what modern neuroscience and genetics tell us. The following is technical but worth a scan. (Even psychiatrists could benefit from reviewing it—unlikely). Please read "Meet Some Suicidal Genes," the introduction to the study, "Identification of Potential Blood Biomarkers," and the summary.

The Black Pit

In severe major depression, the accompaniment of neurobiological dysregulation can result in a sort of brain freeze. Certain cognitions (severe negative neuropsychological cognitive content) become set as if in concrete, taking on an extreme intensity and fixity, rising like a gusher from the emotional brain (the limbic system) to flood logical reasoning (largely a cortical function).

Encouraging an individual in the grips of such tenacious cognitions and their beliefs content to simply get on with it, is as logical as informing the water bursting forth from a dam to recede. Such advice, even well-intentioned advice, is like criticizing an individual caught in the flow of rampaging water to just get over it. The cognitions are of an extreme, catastrophic nature. Everything of value—their own positive identity, relationships, occupational status, and health—are being decimated. That they will end up helpless, totally disabled, in a barren state hospital room or dead. To the outsider, this can appear ridiculous, but in the cognitive black pit, it is a reality for the sufferer. The black pit cognitive phenomenon is accompanied by equivalently catastrophic emotions of fear, horror, dread, and profound hopelessness. That is what occurs in severe major depression.

For centuries, most people have questioned why any individual would contemplate suicide, let alone actually do it. Leading sentiments have been that the suicidal suffer from a weakness of will, cowardice, selfishness, and above all, an absence of grit. And such perspectives are still highly prevalent. The treatment for suicidality should be the proverbial pulling oneself up by one's bootstraps, the abjuration of self-pity, and simply forging ahead, getting on with it. Many psychoanalysts-psychiatrists postulate a fundamental weakness of ego (essentially synonymous with willpower). People with that defect therefore succumb to negative emotional drives.

But some researchers (not psychoanalyst-psychiatrists) have dug a little deeper into other possible causes for suicidal behavior, even though psychiatrists have warned them they are wasting valuable government funds meant to promote research on such a timely subject as suicide. Indeed, the psychoanalyst-psychiatrists affirm the causes of suicide have long been ascertained, starting with the pioneering work of Sigmund Freud and his successors. But some people don't listen. They are driven by excessive professional ambition, funding-hunger, and powerful dysfunctional, maladaptive drives characterized by grandiosity, denial, and passive-aggression.

But they persisted in their research to discover the causes of suicide even though it was against the advice of psychiatry, which informed them that the cause of suicide was already established and explained, in grossly oversimplified terms, to help the nonpsychiatric researchers comprehend: suicide is caused by psychodynamic processes, the id "inverting," thereby bombarding the ego, causing it to fracture, coming perilously close to disintegration.

Johanna Reiss

She was born April 4, 1932, in the Netherlands. When she was seven, the Germans occupied the country. It became apparent that Jewish people were in acute danger. Her father located a rural family which agreed to hide Johanna (Annie) and her sister. They remained cooped up in a room for three years, the family being cautious that the Germans never become aware of them, as they, for the act of boarding Jews (two young girls), would also be slaughtered.

And so, these enemies of *Das Grosse Deutsche Reich* (the Great German Empire) somehow survived. After the Germans retreated and Canadian troops liberated them, they were to become part of that tiny minority of survivors of the German continent-wide mass-murder industry. After the war, Annie attempted to pick up her life again in Holland, but her family elected to emigrate to America in the early 1950s.

In America, she got married and had a very productive literary career, authoring several books. *The Upstairs Room*,[33] published in 1972, won several awards, including an American Library Association Children's Book Award. Elie Wiesel had commented *The Upstairs Room* was as important an accounting of the horrors of WWII for these two Jewish young ladies as Anne Frank's *The Diary of a Young Girl*. In January 2009, Annie's book *A Hidden Life* was published, in which the author again confronted the tragedy of her childhood but also that of her husband's suicide.

The Upstairs Room Summary

Annie relates in detail her experiences when the Germans invaded and occupied the Netherlands. She was seven when it occurred in 1938. She was listening to the radio with her parents. She remembered that they seemed upset. A man called Hitler had invaded their country. Subsequently her parents labored under an incredibly detailed, expanding list of restrictions and oppressions, a monument to German efficiency and capacity for exquisite detail (museeholocauste.ca). Her father was abruptly fired and

---

33   https:/www.supersummary.com/the-upstairs-room/summary.

remained unemployed; her aunt and uncle departed for America, but her mother refused to consider that, maintaining the belief that Jews would be safe. By the time the situation had become desperate, it was too late for her father to make travel arrangements, so he quickly had to look for places to hide. He decided he would split the family, hiding Annie and her sister separately from the rest of the family. He found an accommodating rural family. Annie and her sister were comfortable there, but their hosts, who were indeed taking a serious risk by boarding them, soon requested that the girls find an alternate placement. Their father did locate another rural family, the Oostervelds, who were willing to harbor his daughters. They were confined, however, to a single small room, not allowed to leave. And they spent three years thus cooped up. But they survived. There were two close shaves. On one occasion, when Annie was hiding behind a closet, a German soldier was standing directly in front of her hiding place. On another, she was descending a flight of stairs when a German soldier possibly got a glimpse of her.

After the war, Annie returned to Holland. Her family, in the early 1950s, made the decision to emigrate to America. Years later, she travelled back to Holland with her children, showing them where she had hidden. However, it did reawaken posttraumatic aspects she had experienced after the war. She had episodes of prolonged fear and repeated urges to hide. Most of all, even though she had lived through the experiences, she could not get over the stress of being hunted like vermin, like a rat, with the intention of imminent extermination courtesy of the gentle German exterminators.

She developed an interest in the topic of suicide when her husband took his own life early in their marriage.

Books About Suicide
(recommended by Johanna Reiss)

In 1969, while Johanna Reiss was writing her memoir, *The Upstairs Room*, her American husband, Jim, committed suicide. For "Five Books," she selected five on that topic to review: *Remembering Denny*, by Calvin Trillin; *Darkness Visible* by William Styron; *Night,* by Elie Wiesel; *Night Falls Fast* by Kay Redfield Jamison; and *The Savage God* by Al Alvarez. She was asked why she chose her first book, *Remembering Denny.* Her husband, Jim, and the subject of the book, Denny, both went to Yale. They were so similar, excellent students whose peers thought they would excel in their future endeavors. Denny was a Rhodes Scholar; Jim had a Fulbright[34]. And yet they ended up thinking they were failures, probably undone by perfectionistic expectations. She was asked why Jim was working in retail rather than as a writer or journalist. His father interacted with him only minimally. While serving in the army, he was impressed by a superior officer who became a father figure. The officer had formed the opinion that Jim might do well as a businessman, so he gave up a full scholarship at Yale Law School, instead matriculating at Harvard Business School. He did not have a scholarship there. Annie never felt that it was the right choice for him. He had a gentle soul and lacked skills to maneuver in the business world. Jim, like Denny, became more withdrawn. He ended up, like Denny, "in his own closed box."

William Styron, the author of *Sophie's Choice,* in his sixties, suffered from a "terrible, terrible depression," which was the subject of *Darkness Visible.* Ms. Reiss commented that, unlike Jim, Styron was immobilized by his depression, hardly being able to get out of bed. Somehow Jim had continued in his routines. Styron, on the edge of suicide, just happened to hear Brahms's *Alto Rhapsody,* which brought back memories of how his mother used to sing it to him. Somehow, that had a life-saving effect. He woke up his wife to take him to the hospital.

Mrs. Reiss reflected, "What strikes me is that in many cases, if people had been able to ask for help…their suicides could have been prevented." Jim's suicide occurred forty years previously. She didn't know if he realized he needed help. "There was a lot of stigma attached to going to ask for help." Unlike Styron's situation, she "had no inkling something was wrong."

---

34 https://fivebook.com/best-books/suicide-Johanna-Reiss/pgs. 1-2.

She read in the Jamison book, *Night Falls Fast,* that thirty thousand fatal suicides occur yearly (actually, it's over forty-five thousand) and half a million make a consequential suicide attempt. Jamison attempted suicide at age twenty-eight. Jamison describes suicide as "a response to an unendurable level of mental pain." They do it because it seems to them to be, at the time, the only reasonable option available to get rid of the terrible mental anguish they are experiencing. To the outsider not experiencing such subjective anguish, the suicidal behavior appears irrational. The intense dysphoria is reflected in suicide notes. "I couldn't bear the pain any longer."

She was asked to discuss Elie Wiesel's book *Night,* how the inmates in the concentration camps coped with that utter barbarism courtesy of the Germans. The inmates' consuming focus was to obtain any crust of bread they could lay their hands on. Elie Wiesel briefly considered executing himself on the barbed-wire fence but was inhibited by the thought he couldn't desert his father, also an inmate.

Overall, there were fewer suicides than one would anticipate given the hideous, ghastly circumstances that had been so refined by German ingenuity. She commented that if there is a reason not to attempt suicide, it's that someone or something would be far worse off because of it. That can be a powerful deterrent, but not always. Sometimes the emotional pain and the associated suicidal ruminations are so powerful they extinguish any countervailing thoughts of the consequences for loved, significant others. Johanna Reiss coined the term "a closed box," which describes the impenetrability of the suicidal ruminations in some individuals.

Her last book, *The Savage God,* was written by the English poet Al Alvarez. He began his book by discussing the poet Sylvia Plath, arguing that suicide is frequent particularly in "the creative world": Sylvia Plath, Ernest Hemingway, Van Gogh, Primo Levi, and so many others. Alvarez avers that "even though suicide seems like a solution in the minds of those who do it, actually, it is a form of failure, just as a divorce is a failure at some level."

For Mrs. Reiss, for a long time, she wasn't able to mourn Jim's loss. She was fixated on raising her two daughters "because I had to be strong for my daughters. I had to get these kids through it…I had to bring them up…I didn't want to be a miserable mother who wails and sits and weeps…I didn't begin dealing with Jim's suicide, really, until I began writing *A Hidden Life*, which is why it took me so long, because it was a very hard thing to do."

Meet Some Suicidal Genes

But it may not be so simple that suicide is simply something we do to ourselves, implying we always have an option to "snap out" of that state of mind. Could it be that there are actually genes associated with suicide? Such genes serve as "biomarkers" for patients at high risk for suicide by means of a blood sample, similar to how a blood sample is used to diagnose diabetes.

The researchers presented their latest laboratory research findings to the Psychoanalytic-Psychiatric all-inclusive annual meeting. The psychiatrists had definitively ruled out the possibility of genes playing a role in "mental illness" (it's just common sense; how can a microscopic gene possibly play a role in the basic cause of "mental" illness, deeply buried unconscious conflicts?). But they agreed to listen.

The following study was dismissed by the Psychoanalytic-psychiatric research committee, as they rejected the idea that deep emotional conflicts have any association with such tiny entities as genes—microscopic particles, after all, which could not possibly be the structures from which such complex unconscious drives and conflicts could emanate. The committee would investigate the possibility of the existence of "mental" genes, however.

Identification of Potential Blood Biomarkers Associated with Suicide in Major Depressive Disorder. Firoza Mamdani, Et Al.

Translational Psychiatry 12, Article number 159 (2022)

Hopefully, at some point in the not-too-distant future, blood tests will be used to diagnose M.D.D.(major depressive disorder) as they are used to diagnose diabetes. And more specifically, a blood test which can diagnose suicidality in a subpopulation of patients with M.D.D., distinguishing them from those who aren't.

Many patients who are serious suicidal risks do not disclose their despair and hopelessness, leaving little opportunity to intervene until the terminal event has occurred. Currently, a simple blood test in the research phase could identify them, opening up an opportunity for an intervention to interrupt the suicidal sequence.

In the introduction, the authors comment there are nearly fifty thousand completed suicides annually in spite of current interventions and treatments. M.D.D. is by far the most common cause of suicide. The ultimate objective of their study was "to identify changes in gene expression associated with suicide in brain and blood of people with M.D.D.," for development of biomarkers for suicide, which ultimately would provide the basis for blood tests used in clinical settings. Samples were collected from two experimental groups and a control group: (MDD-S), M.D.D. patients who died by suicide; (MDD-NS), M.D.D. patients who died from other causes, and non-psychiatric controls. Fourteen genes significantly differentiated MDD-S from MDD-NS in the blood, and twenty-one genes from one region of the cortex, the DLPPC (dorsal lateral prefrontal cortex). "Developing a suicide biomarker signature in blood could help healthcare professionals to identify subjects at high risk for suicide" (even without interviewing them).

"Mental" Illness

So-called "mental" illnesses have been "dichotomized" away from all the other illnesses human beings are subject to by psychiatry. They are classified as entirely different from "physical" illnesses. They have their own diagnostic manual, *The Diagnostic and Statistical Manual of Mental Disorders, Fifth Edition, DSM-5*, published by the American Psychiatric Association. No other medical specialty has so obviously separated itself in that manner and degree from all the other medical specialties that are included in the general Manual of Diagnostic Classification, ICD-10-CM/PCS-Mapping. So, this is a startling, clear division: "mental" vs. "physical." And this has heavily colored how we think about these two categories.

Now psychiatrists consider themselves erudite in the matter of subconscious and unconscious processes of the mind, yet they continue to cleave to this strict dichotomous classification, so nearly everybody—the press, the media, most physicians, and the general public—does the same. We automatically do so, generally meaning no harm. The dichotomy is so ingrained that it infuses everyone's thinking, and we judge accordingly. But there is harm!

Psychiatrists, those masters of unconscious symbolism, have evidently never subjected themselves to the following exercise: Draw a line midway on a page. As a preliminary, let your mind relax. Enter a state in which your thoughts just wander so you can free-associate. Avoid critical thinking. Now write down all the words, phrases, and unconscious beliefs about mentally ill people. Repeat for so-called "physical" illness on the other half of the page. Continue until no further thoughts come.

Actually, this author doubts the average psychiatrist can honestly report this exercise. If they try (doubtful), it would induce too much "unconscious conflict" (which, of course, is their explanation for the *causes* of so-called "mental" illnesses).

There is an entirely separate health care system for the "mental cases," the "mental health care system," and so there should be for these weird people (who would cause too much disruption in the general health care system!). And for these suffering people (are they really suffering or just weak-willed?), is it helpful to them to label them "mental cases?" Possibly they are really in discomfort. So, does it make them more comfortable to do so?

So, psychiatry still pitches its "mental" illness categorization into the third decade of the twenty-first century. (Presumably they could continue to do so until the twenty-second century?)

The Mental Illness Classification

Is there really such a thing as "mental" illness? What is the origin of the terminology? What is the effect of this classification? Is it time to change it in this new era of imaging technology and in-depth laboratory research on neurotransmitters and other aspects of detailed dysregulation of intimate physical brain systems, particularly the process of elevated apoptosis in the brain (hyperapoptosis)? Is there really such a thing as "mental" illness? Certainly "mental" symptoms exist and are real, inducing discomfort, misery, and disability. But the brain is not the only body-organ from which "mental" symptoms can originate. A variety of medical and neurological diseases can also present with or be manifested by "mental" symptoms, but it's only the brain which is shoved off into a stereotyped "mental" classification, a second tier of human illness, if there are prominent emotional, cognitive, or behavioral symptoms. They are then draped in a special cloak of stigma and humiliation.

The "mental" illness/"mental" health terminology arose in the early twentieth century, long before the advent of technologically sophisticated imaging and laboratory research. Freud himself, by training a neurologist, spent a great deal of effort to discover the physical causes for his dawning awareness of so-called "mental" symptoms but came up empty-handed. Even the ancients knew this particular set of human ailments existed, but on inspecting the brains of such individuals, they found no particular evidence of physical causes that they could see on gross inspection. Freud, however, endowed with a particularly fertile imagination, proceeded to construct a psychological system that could explain "mental" symptoms. One wonders, if he could revisit in this era, apart from culture shock, whether he would take like a duck to water to the data from both imaging studies and the modern laboratory. That would really be a worthy "thought experiment," to speculate how he might react! But those who succeeded Freud, by and large, lacked his genius, and over the next century continued to uncritically adhere to a psychological model of causation: deep unconscious conflict, a brain ridden with intrusive motivations and drives, controlled by powerful hostility and sexual impulses. These are the beliefs of current psychoanalysts, who are largely psychiatrists. But some "mental" health professionals, though few psychiatrists, have broken that mold, and a number of evidence-based psychotherapies, i.e., cognitive behavioral therapy, has been developed and utilized.

A brief discussion of "evidence." What does "evidence-based" mean? For therapeutic procedures in general medicine, psychiatry and psychology, the gold standard of efficacy of a treatment is the double-blind, randomized, controlled study in which maximum scientific effort is made to compare treatments to each other and "placebos" (sugar-pill treatment), keeping out all variables that could interfere with an accurate determination of the true efficacy of the treatment or treatments, which need to be evaluated for benefit and safety (or lack thereof). All adverse effects must be noted. A "meta-analysis" occurs when a number of valid studies have accumulated that demonstrate together that a treatment or treatments give consistent, reliable results.

It must be noted that so-called "mental" health treatments are held to the same standards in studies and meta-analysis as the treatments for "physical" illnesses. So, as we continue through the twenty-first century, should we just perpetuate the "mental illness/mental health" terminology? How does the current system of labeling and classification, so sanctioned by psychiatry, actually affect potential patients or actual patients? Does it facilitate their motivation to be identified as "mental cases" and to arrange for "mental health" treatment? Are they more motivated to continue in whatever "mental" health treatment they become involved with and to comply with the recommendations for such treatment? At this juncture, 50-60 percent of people with troubling "mental" symptoms never seek treatment for their symptoms, sometimes ramping up visitations with family physicians or internists, or more likely just suffering from nonspecific complaints and successive difficulties in their lives tied to their "mental" symptoms. Even those who meet the challenge of accepting the label "mental case" may enter into a state of confusion, in addition to their symptoms and suffering, because of the diffuse nature of the so-called "mental health care system" and its varied flock of "mental" health providers. This can be very costly to those with serious illness (in which hyperapoptosis is most likely occurring). And as their symptoms progress, and they enter into a state of decline either rapidly or slowly, seen or unseen, they don't know what hit them.

"Prevention" is a concept of great importance in medicine. Everyone is aware of the need to prevent epidemics or, if unable to do that, to reduce the spread of a disease in a population, or, if that isn't entirely feasible, to reduce symptoms and disability as much as possible. In the so-called "mental health care system," none of these levels of prevention can even be brought to bear on the 50-60 percent of those suffering from so-called "mental" illness because they never seek treatment. For the other 40-50 percent, treatment is brought to bear late, is not appropriate for a patient's level of symptoms, or is administered erratically.

Well, what has changed in our knowledge of brain pathology and so-called "mental" illnesses?

Apoptosis and Hyperapoptosis

Is any illness in which there is an abnormal rate of dying of brain cells (neurons) just a "mental" problem? Apoptosis is a normal physical brain process but also, in certain brain diseases, can become excessive, in which case brain cells start dying at accelerated rates. Quite obviously, the more that occurs, the more brain tissue diminishes, and in turn, the brain actually shrinks in size. And accelerated APOPTOSIS occurs obviously in neurological diseases such as stroke (cerebral vascular accidents), multiple sclerosis, and Parkinson's and Alzheimer's disease.

What Is Apoptosis?

Talk about the ingenuity of Mother Nature. How do you manage trillions of cells, eliminating the ones that have defects or need to be trimmed like a piece of fat off a steak, while simultaneously sustaining a sufficient degree of control so a normal, optimal number of neurons are preserved? It's a delicate balance, a fine-tuning that must occur. And apoptosis is a head-spinning, complicated process!

This author will attempt a simplification while simultaneously, to some degree, conveying the complexity. Why bother to review this topic? It is the main process that can lead to excessive degrees of neuron death as part of a process not necessarily precipitated by some external cause or injury. In the case of the brain, excessive apoptosis results in actual shrinkage of the brain as neuron death is rapidly accelerated. Yes, progressive elimination of neurons! That's *us* being whittled away!

And no one could deny apoptosis is a "physical" phenomenon! Some examples follow.

Apoptosis (and Hyper)

Apoptosis is programmed cell death, which leads to the elimination of body cells (including neurons) in a fashion that avoids creating a toxicity that could damage other cells or tissues in the vicinity. It is critical to health maintenance because it refines tissues and organs. In the central nervous system, it more or less "sculpts" the architecture of the brain. Cells which are undergoing apoptosis have character-istic changes in shape. The cell membranes develop blebs, and the cell shrinks. The DNA in the nucleus fragments. The cell, however, does not disintegrate, scattering its toxic debris into the intercellular spaces, which would damage other tissue. Instead, it breaks into por-tions called apoptotic bodies, which are engulfed by specialized cells, phagocytes, that destroy those bodies in a "clean" fashion.

Apoptosis utilizes some fierce-sounding agents. There are the caspases, specialized proteins that participate in the apoptosis process. One particular caspase initiates apoptosis (actually, there are several). Then the "executioner" caspases do the murdering, "indiscriminate-ly" degrading the proteins of the cells, which are then loaded into the apoptotic bodies prior to phagocytosis (in which specialized blood cells ingest and destroy them). Dysregulated apoptosis is associated with a wide variety of diseases. Insufficient apoptosis results in un-controlled proliferation of cells, which occurs in cancers. Excessive apoptosis causes atrophy of the organ in which it is occurring. A num-ber of factors termed "Fas" receptors and caspases speed up apoptosis. Others, the Bcl-2 "family" of proteins, inhibit it. And controlling all of this is a host of particular genes.

Factors that can initiate apoptosis activate the "death-inducing signaling complex" (DISC), in which cell-surface death receptors are activated by external circumstances like heat, radiation, nutrient deprivation, viral infection, insufficient oxygen (hypoxia), and excessive calcium. Once apoptosis is triggered, it can proceed by complex mechanisms in the "intrinsic" or "extrinsic" pathways (which require pages of explanation to describe in detail). Just to give the flavor (no need to understand, just see how complex and physical the process is), examples of molecules involved include TNF-alpha, TNFR1, TNFR2, the binding of TNF-alpha to TNFR1, TRADD (THF receptor-associated death domain), Fas-associated death domain protein (FADD), CTAP1/2, (which inhibits TNF-a), TRAF2, FLIP, caspase-8, death receptors DRJ and DR5, protein TRAIL, and we could go on!

The main point: no one in their right mind would describe apoptosis as a "mental" process due to deep unconscious conflicts!

For the purposes of this discussion, we are concerned with up-regulated apoptosis, or "hyperapoptosis," which results if the controls on cell death become defective. An assortment of diseases can arise. These include neurological illnesses such as Parkinson's or Alzheimer's, Human Immunodeficiency Virus (HIV and AIDS), and other viral infections, even canine (dog) diseases (Canine distemper virus-COV).

In the case of the brain, hyperapoptosis causes accelerated neuron cell death per unit time, resulting in the diminishment of the size of brain regions, associated symptom intensification, and loss of functions. This occurs in Parkinson's and Alzheimer's diseases. The loss of cognitive and/or motor capabilities is progressive. The latest neuroscientific research has demonstrated that hyperapoptosis also occurs in the so-called "mental" illnesses, schizophrenia, bipolar disorder, and major, recurrent depression.

Brain Research in the Modern Era

Sigmund Freud just gave up. He, a trained neurologist, could not identify any physical abnormalities underlying "mental" symptoms and constructed instead an ingenious system of "mental" phenomena as the causative agents. He would probably salivate if he knew of the

THE INCREDIBLE SHRINKING BRAIN

existence of our new technologies, sophisticated imaging techniques of the brain (MRI, PET), and the laboratory research that has discovered numerous neurotransmitters and other molecules and hormones which, it is now known, are associated with so-called "mental" disorders. But in his era, it made sense to separate so-called "mental" disorders from "physical" disorders, as the former seemed to exist without discernible physical etiology. And we still live with that dichotomy, which this author has labeled "the treacherous dichotomy" because it isolates "mental" diseases from all others, which are categorized as "physical," implying that somehow, they aren't as important or serious, resulting in an automatic demotion, often unconscious, in the minds of the public.

The New Sciences: Imaging and Laboratory

Sigmund Freud never had the chance to review the data that has come forth from imaging and neuroscientific research, and he couldn't have had a detailed scientific understanding of dysregulated apoptosis.

Most people know that in serious neurological diseases, stroke, brain cancer, Alzheimer's disease, and Parkinson's disease, parts of the brain are damaged, and that must mean people with such diseases have lost brain tissue and therefore brain cells (neurons). That is plain common sense: that neurological diseases are obviously physical diseases.

Imaging Studies: What do they demonstrate about the so-called "mental" illnesses? Are they just caused by "mental" problems and unconscious conflicts? Is there really such a thing, a "mental" disease caused by "mental" conflicts? Do "mental" diseases actually exist as distinct, actual diseases? But the stigmatizing label is perpetuated by psychiatry. We can review a selection of imaging studies of "mental cases."

But first, for the sake of comparison, let's visit an obvious "physical" neurological disease caused by deficient oxygen in the brain, "Apoptotic Mechanisms After Cerebral Ischemia." (Broughton, PhD, Reutens, MD and Sobey PhD, ahajournals.org, Sept. 13, 2021.)

We'll also review briefly apoptosis occurring in multiple sclerosis and Parkinson's disease.

Ischemic diseases (deprivation of oxygen to the brain sections affected) are caused by the cutoff of blood supply due to the blockage of a vessel transporting oxygenated blood to the brain. Where oxygen cutoff is complete, neurons disintegrate (necrosis). Around that core death zone is another, larger zone of cells, which, instead of undergoing total destruction immediately, destroys itself in that very orderly death program, apoptosis. That hyperapoptotic region is labeled the "ischemic penumbra." And in that area, vast numbers of neurons are committing suicide.

In the neurological disease multiple sclerosis, as inflammation and hyperapoptosis progress, a whole host of neurological symptoms follow: fatigue, numbness, loss of balance, paralysis of eye muscles, double vision, partial blindness, general muscle spasticity, vertigo, abnormal speech, and impaired swallowing—obviously a wide variety of challenging physical symptoms.

Parkinson's disease is another serious neurological illness in which hyperapoptosis is the major cause of neuron (brain cell) death, and as hyperapoptosis accelerates, symptoms are exacerbated. Body movements slow down, facial expressions become frozen or "masked," falls occur frequently due to postural instability, extremities become stiff and rigid, tremors increase, and gaits become unstable, along with general decreased body movement. A dementia-type syndrome can occur, which hastens death. A primary cause is a shortage of the neurotransmitter dopamine, as the neurons which produce it suicide via hyperapoptosis.

As an interesting sidenote, hyperapoptosis has been determined to be the main cause of death of immune cells in human immunodeficiency virus (HIV). Starting in the early 1980s, HIV was nearly always fatal until the introduction of new medications. The cause of the illness was hyperaptotic cell-death of critical infection-fighting blood cells, CD4-T and CD8-1 cells.

The preceding examples all occur when apoptosis is upregulated (hyperapoptosis), so obviously, it's strictly a physical bodily process. In terms of "mental" problems, one would never anticipate that this precise program of neuron cell death would be implicated, that hyperapoptosis could even be occurring.

Industrious researchers (not psychiatrists) were completely ignorant of the deep "mental" conflicts that psychiatrists claim cause "mental" illness, but they were incentivized to conduct imaging studies on so-called "mental" cases to obtain grant money, which pays their salaries and expedites the publication of the imaging studies that enhance their professional reputations. Thousands of imaging studies of "real" physical illnesses already existed. Where to turn for new subjects? Well, "mental cases," it was thought, would open up a new area in which to undertake imaging studies—if nothing else, to demonstrate the absence of physical brain damage that is so obviously apparent in neurological diseases. Imaging research on "mental cases" would extend the reach of imaging technology even if there were no demonstrable physical abnormalities in the examined brains of such "mental cases." So, a new industry arose, imaging the brains of people with schizophrenia, bipolar disorder, and severe unipolar major depression. (Fortunately, the researchers did not consult in depth with psychiatrists, who would have counseled them not to waste their funds and time. Deep, unconscious conflicts cannot be visualized, only becoming apparent in deep psychoanalytic psychotherapy.)

Nevertheless, the imaging studies proceeded. "Hippocampal correlates of depression in healthy elderly adults," Ezzati, et al, PMCID: 239 398 71, PMC4018740, DOI: 10 1002/hipo.22185.

The hippocampus is a major structure in the brain, located on both sides, left and right. It is not physically imposing, but it is extremely important for memory and cognitive functions. It registers information from the environment in short-term memory and also transforms the short-term memory into long-term memory. It is also responsible for spatial memory, facilitating movement in three-dimensional space.

Operative in the hippocampi is N-acetyl aspartate. It plays an important role in memory. Creatine (CR) is a waste product. Patients with clinical depression were studied with (1) complex imaging procedures and (2) in-depth psychological testing. Hippocampal N-acetyl aspartate ratio was abnormal (NAA/CR), with significantly diminished NAA to CR. The findings showed that both lower hippocampal volumes and a lower level of hippocampal N-acetyl aspartate predicted decreased, impaired memory ability.

(1) 4-T MRI, proton magnetic resonance spectroscopy. Magnetic Resonance Imaging 12(3): 457.

(2) Cved Selective Reminding Test – Immediate Recall, Wechsler Memory Scale, Romsed; Trail Making Test Parts A and B.

Question: Could a mere "mental" problem cause such diminished hippocampi?

Further Imaging Studies and Research Findings in Major Depressive Disorder (MDD)

The author has tried to simplify the results, but for readers who do not wish to read through the material, there follows a brief summary.

Summary Studies in MDD

Patients with a diagnosis of MDD have smaller hippocampi (atrophied) and lower levels of metabolites, N-acetyl aspartate, lactate, and choline, in contrast to H.C. (healthy controls). The hippocampi facilitate working memory and learning ability. Lactate is a fuel in neurons that is important for normal interneuron signaling. Choline is a component of acetylcholine, a critical neurotransmitter. Also, there is mitochondrial dysfunction, which leads to abnormal glycolysis, impairing use of glucose, a fuel. Oxygen utilization is reduced. Neuroplasticity is deficient, resulting in decreased capacity to form new neuronal connections (synapses) in response to environmental challenges.

But according to psychiatry, psychoanalytic psychotherapy will be corrective for these "mental" problems.

Details of the Studies are in the Appendix

Well, our researchers (non-psychiatrists), excited by their results, set up a meeting with psychiatrists at a prominent psychoanalytic institute. The psychiatrists listened politely, but they knew psychopathology was not caused by mere physical processes in the brain. How totally mechanistic and naïve! There was possibly one small area of agreement (possibly), the issue of depth or deepness. The hippocampi certainly are situated deep in the brain, so they do have that commonality with deeply buried unconscious conflicts.

After the meeting, our researchers retreated back to their laboratories, rather forlorn in mood. Could they ever convince their psychiatrist friends with the accumulating neuroscientific evidence, which demonstrates that actual abnormal physical mechanisms in the brain that are etiological in schizophrenia, bipolar disorder, and severe major depression are really more scientifically validated than psychoanalytic theory? (It is said that outdated theories only die when their proponents do).

Imaging Studies before and after ECT (electroconvulsive treatment)

What is Electroconvulsive Therapy? (ECT)

It was introduced in Italy in 1938 for the treatment of severe illness. In the next ten-fourteen years, it became clear that it was a useful treatment, ameliorating serious symptoms, including suicidality, and it did not attract that much attention from the media.

Then *One Flew over the Cuckoo's Nest* appeared in theaters in 1975, based on a novel of the same name by Ken Kesey. The film starred Jack Nicholson playing a criminal in a penitentiary who malingers having a mental illness so he will be transferred to the mental ward of the prison, which he believes will be more lenient. Being the sociopath he is, it isn't long before he serially misbehaves and next is "treated" with electroshock therapy, administered brutally. He is held standing against the wall by force. The two paddles are applied to his right and left forehead as he grimaces and squirms. Next, he has a violent grand mal convulsion. Finally, he is carried out, limp. There has been brain damage. He behaves as if he has been lobotomized. This is how the general public was introduced to the treatment, the name of which, "electroshock," is consistent with the portrayal in the film.

———

Source: Principles and Practice of Psychopharmacology; Janicak, Davis, Preskorn, and Ayd, Jr. Lippincott Williams & Wilkins.

The authors note, clearly, that electroconvulsive therapy (ECT) has stood the test of time. They review past problems associated with it, but in modern medical facilities, it is now administered in a highly structured fashion for severe illnesses in which pharmacological approaches (attempted trials with antidepressants, antipsychotics, lithium, or other mood stabilizers and various combinations used together) have not diminished severe suffering and symptoms. It is especially efficacious and rapidly acting for high-risk patients who are acutely suicidal or are undergoing rapid physical deterioration. It specifically relieves severe mood distress, severe insomnia, severe lack of appetite, general loss of interest in relevant activities, and severe blocking of the capacity to experience any sense of pleasure or satisfaction (anhedonia), a pervasive boredom and tediousness coloring all experiences.

The procedure is quite gentle when administered in a modern medical center. Like any other surgical procedure, the patient is asleep during the treatment. There are barely any untoward body movements. The patient awakens in the recovery room with nurses in attendance. Usually, two or three treatments are given in a week, over two or three weeks. Patients are relieved of horrible distress, able to cheer up and again carry on socially.

Imaging studies of patients who have had ECT have been useful in quantifying the physical parameters of brain areas before and after a course of it. It is remarkable how organized psychiatry still classifies the illnesses they treat as "mental," even though the *purely physical* treatment is so highly effective. It's as if neurologists treating neurological illnesses also with pharmacology, or operative procedures, had decided to declare that neurological illnesses are "mental."

Summary of Studies in MDD After ECT

A very important brain circuit connecting five brain regions regulates mood-state, emotions, and motivational drive (reward systems) and contains the brain's pleasure center. The circuit also plays a role in addictions. After ECT treatment, two important components, the striatum and palladium, were significantly increased in volume, which did not occur in matched controls. It was postulated that the birth of new neurons had occurred. Another disease, HIV-AIDS, like in MDD, leads to smaller hippocampi. Is the latter "physical" and the former merely "mental?"

The details of the studies are in the appendix.

Introduction:
Bipolar Disorder

Bipolar disorder is another "mental" illness in the mood category. There are approximately three million "mental cases" with this illness in the United States. For a "mental" problem, the symptoms can be severe, resulting in painful disruptions of daily routines in important life areas. Some people with this illness can become "manic," running wild. They won't even listen when told to "snap out of it!" Perhaps the most direct way to encourage them to choose to snap out of it was the approach used in the Middle Ages: placement in the village stockades, whipping, and imprisonment in lunatic asylums. Unfortunately, the Enlightenment in Europe curtailed those effective therapies!

The task of the psychiatrist in treating bipolar disorder can become a burden because they resist the intensive psychoanalytic interpretations of the psychiatrists, which would extirpate the deep emotional conflicts, which, in turn, would cure their symptoms. But many psychiatrists suspect that patients don't have any deep emotional conflicts, but are stubborn, sociopathic individuals who thrive on chaos, refusing to snap out of it.

But then, bless modern science and the researchers employing the new technologies, imaging techniques, and laboratory research. At last, there has been a rational inquiry.

Evidently, even children can have "mental" symptoms, and there has been a running speculation about just how deep their emotional conflicts could be. One opinion is that the deep emotional conflicts predate birth by several months and therefore are really, really deep. This issue may never be settled, as no one to date has been able to employ psychoanalysis on an embryo or a fetus.

Children, however, have been studied with in vivo (meaning the children were alive) proton magnetic resonance spectroscopy (which can actually detect chemicals in the brain). The children in one study had mood symptoms and a family history of bipolar disorder. Particular attention was paid to the scans of the prefrontal cortex (the folded areas of the outer surface, in the front of the brain) and the cerebellar vermis (that's not a worm but a structure in the lower rear of the brain, the outer part looking like spaghetti). They determined, in contrast to the healthy children who served as comparisons, that the affected children had "neurochemical abnormalities" in these two structures, such as decreased N-acetyl aspartate and creatinine and phosphocreatine. (Don't worry about what they are, but they are associated with disturbed metabolism in these two important brain areas). The researchers concluded the children had the same neurochemical abnormalities as adults with bipolar disorder.

Arachidonic acid was first detected in the brain in 1922. Due to modern brain imaging and capacity to detect important molecules in the brain, arachidonic acid signaling can be measured with positron emission tomography. Arachidonic acid signals regulate neuroinflammation and excitotoxicity, which, if excessive—meaning that is there are abnormally high cascades of the signaling—can result in rampant neuronal injury and death. It is of note that certain medications used to treat bipolar disorder, lithium, carbamazepine, and valproate, down-regulate arachidonic acid signaling. Note: How can such a clearly damaging physical process be subsumed under the category "mental?" The bigoted belief that "mental" patients should "snap out of it," that "mental" cases have deficient willpower, is far older than the neuroscientific findings on arachidonic acid signaling and far outweighs it in influence on the public mind. And if one could query most psychiatrists, it is doubtful they are informed about arachidonic acid signaling. A future prospect is that the phenomenon of arachidonic acid signaling could lead to new imaging techniques and novel therapeutic agents. (Could that have more potential to relieve suffering than the psychiatrists shooting out those brilliant, incisive psychiatric interpretations to cure deep emotional conflicts in the unconscious in intensive, psychoanalytically oriented deep psychotherapy, one to four therapy sessions weekly, for two to ten years?)

And individuals who have bipolar illness, of course, die, but at ages ten-fifteen years younger than people not afflicted. (Suicide does not account for this diminished longevity. There may be something "physical" going on.) There is only one positive aspect to this shortened span of life: scientists don't have to wait as long to do postmortem autopsies.

Bipolar Disorder
(Multiple Physical Dysregulations in the Brain)

Note on the following text on bipolar disorder[35]. It is highly technical but has not been placed in the appendix. It is meant to illustrate the complex, intricate, *physical* causes of the illness. It is a "neurological-like illness. One possible way to reclassify it is to call it a *neuriatric* illness, employing the same root as *neur*ology. That would be a start in rejecting once and for all the stigmatizing treatment-avoidance cause of the archaic *mental* classification. Unfortunately, organized psychiatry will dig in its heels, as the great bulk of their income derives from what is a "mental" therapy: traditional psychiatric weekly, full session, psychotherapy. The psychotherapy can be a useful treatment, but not if it inhibits the replacing of the "mental" referencing of these illnesses with scientifically more accurate, less stigmatizing nomenclature.

---

35 Altered expression of apoptotic ratio and synaptic markers in post mortem brain from bipolar patients. Hyung-Wook Kim, Stanley Rapoport, Jaga deesch Rao. Neurobial. Dis. 2010 Marc. 37(3) 596-603.

Approach to the text on bipolar disorder for the reader: for those willing to plow through the entire text, please proceed. Again, it is not necessary to understand everything, but instead to gain a notion of the multiple *physical* brain dysregulations causative of bipolar disorder. (It is obviously not a "mental" problem, as psychiatry has classified it.)

Otherwise, just scan through, but try to read: On Apoptosis and hyperapoptosis; what is a review article?; and the authors have written; so, what are the consequences?; One thing is truly amazing; multiple consistent and convergent evidence; the authors conclude their review in summary.

Altered expression of apoptotic ratio and synaptic markers in postmortem brain from bipolar disorder patients. Hyung-Wook Kim, Stanley Rapoport, Jagadeesch Rao. Neurobiol. Dis. 2010 Mar. 37 (3) 596-603. In the abstract it states:

"Bipolar disorder is a progressive psychiatric disorder characterized by recurrent changes of mood and is associated with cognitive decline."

This implies an association with detrimental "physical" brain processes, i.e., hyperapoptosis, brain atrophy, etc. How could a "mental" problem or deep unconscious conflicts result in cognitive decline? That doesn't sound logical or scientific—or, if you will, such a belief may itself be a sign of a "mental" problem.

The researchers were testing if excitotoxic neuroinflammation, upregulated arachidonic cascade signaling, and brain atrophy were implicated in bipolar disorder.

Brief glossary

1. Arachidonic Acid (AA) signaling or cascades. It regulates neuroinflammation and excitotoxicity.
2. Neuroinflammation. An inflammatory response is triggered by infections, traumatic brain injury, toxic metabolites, or autoimmunity; provokes hyperapoptosis, or neurons are directly destroyed.

3. Excitotoxicity. It refers to the overactivity of glutamate receptors, which, in turn, causes nerve cell damage or death (apoptosis), or neurons are directly destroyed.

4. Postmortem study. Carried out by pathologists using laboratory studies to determine what illnesses were the cause of death.

5. Synapse. The junction between nerve cells, consisting of a microscopic gap through which neurotransmitters pass between neurons.

6. Brain atrophy. A shrinking of the brain caused by loss of cells. Symptoms of significant brain atrophy: progressive intellectual impairment leading to dementia, seizures, aphasias, loss of production of and understanding of language.

7. Glutamate: Excessive levels of this excitatory neurotransmitter overstimulates the glutamate/NMDA receptors, resulting in excessive apoptosis or direct death of neurons.

Reminder: the author is using the scientific words employed in the studies. The point is *not* to understand the terms, but to absorb how "physical" the terminology is! (Not an "Oedipus complex" to be seen.)

Apoptosis

In the Discussion" section of this clarifying article, the dysregulation of apoptosis is described through its mechanisms. There are biomolecules that suppress apoptosis or enhance it. A group of proteins, proapoptic factors, upregulate apoptosis. For the record, they are Bax, BAD, and active (caspase3). An alternative group of proteins downregulate it. These are also called neurotrophic proteins, Bel-2 and BDNF (brain-derived neurotrophic factor). It is the ratio of Bax/Bel-2 that decides if neurons live or die. The process of hyperapoptosis is set off by increased arachidonic acid (AA) signaling, which itself is triggered by an enzyme—for the record, calcium dependent phospholipase A_2 (cPLA$_2$). AA then binds to antiapoptotic proteins, while proapoptotic proteins like BAD are released, displacing neurotrophic proteins (Bel-2, BDNF). This is not a positive development, particularly since BDNF might be called an "angelic" protein because it is so kind and helpful to the brain. It wants neurons to be born (neurogenesis), connect optimally (so we are in possession of our native intelligence), and remain plump and healthy.

The researchers carefully analyzed tissue specimens from the brains of deceased people with bipolar disorder and a similar number of brains from normal controls (with no history of a bipolar diagnosis). There were important differences. The bipolar brains had decreased levels of BDNF in the frontal cortex and increased $cPLA_2$ (which "fires up" AA). They also noted a loss of synaptic integrity in the bipolar brains. As in Alzheimer's disease, a presynaptic marker, synaptophysin, and a postsynaptic marker, drebin, were significantly decreased. This may be associated with cognitive deficits in both disorders.

The authors summarize that the increase of proapoptotic factors and the decrease in antiapoptotic factors are associated with the progression of symptoms and disability in bipolar disorder due to progressing brain atrophy. Mood-stabilizing medications may assist in delaying or preventing this morbid pathology.

What Is a Review Article?

It attempts to summarize the existing scientific knowledge about a given topic.

Integrated Neurobiology of Bipolar Disorder: Vladimir, Maletic and Charles Raisin. Frontiers of Psychiatry, 25 August 2014.

The first thing to note is that there is no mention of deep emotional conflicts or Oedipus conflict to be found.

The authors describe a "vicious cycle" in the matter of the diagnosis and treatment of bipolar disorder. Despite "the significant advances in our understanding of the underlying neurobiology of bipolar disorder," they observe "daunting" clinical challenges. (A brief comment: it is only a minority of psychiatrists who have a working knowledge of the neurobiology or the expertise to establish an accurate, timely diagnosis or to institute timely, comprehensive treatment.) The article notes diagnosis is complex due to possible psychiatric, medical, and neurological comorbidities. (Other psychiatric disorders—ADHD, anxiety, personality and substance-use disorders—can confuse the diagnostic picture). The result is increased disease morbidity and mortality and accentuated suicidality.

People with bipolar disorder carry the burden of increased disease: cardiovascular, cerebral-vascular, metabolic, and endocrinal. The result is condemnation to a significantly shortened and disease-burdened life. They note that successive episodes of illness result in "detectable volumetric changes in the brain that have been frequently associated with deterioration in multiple, functional domains." They state that available pharmacologic interventions are plagued by pronounced adverse effects that often aggravate metabolic status and further compromise cognition in people already struggling in this domain.(That's why an experienced clinical psychopharmacologist will achieve better outcomes.)

The authors are very well-intentioned. Headway is being made in understanding "bipolar disorder based on genetics, etiopathogenesis, pathophysiology and alterations on the cellular and sub-cellular levels." The therapeutic objective is to reverse the autonomic, neuroendocrine, and immune system dysfunctions that are characteristic of the disorder, and which almost certainly contribute to the high degree of medical morbidity in bipolarity." They intend to "finally establish a link between macroscopic and microscopic brain changes and the interaction between multiple genetic factors and life's adversities."

And the authors have written a very sound scientific document. It all sounds quite positive and hopeful. But then, there is the emperor—the one with no clothes—from a folktale by Hans Christian Andersen, "The Emperor's New Clothes." The expression developed to indicate how, when the metaphorical veil falls off, what is exposed is an illusion. The illusion is that in the current so-called "mental health care system," with its confusing array of "mental health" therapists, and the current psychiatric profession, which is obsessed with converting each patient by means of psychoanalytic-type psychotherapy into a new, overhauled emotional specimen (forty-five minutes for each patient, often two-four sessions per week), that 80 percent of patients who need to be evaluated by a psychiatrist ever are. In contrast, neurology, the other specialty overseen by the American Board of Psychiatry and Neurology, can evaluate, diagnose, and treat four times the number of patients in a week. Nonspecialist primary practitioners, meanwhile, fill in for the psychiatrists.

It is an illusion that bipolar patients are receiving, in many instances, the brain treatment they need. The result is the free reign of hyperapoptosis. There is often no means by which the average bipolar patient can ferret out a truly medically qualified psychiatrist. The difference between the average psychiatrist and an experienced psychopharmacologist is arcane knowledge to most. It's a bit of Russian roulette with neurons.

The following is a little of what neuroscience has uncovered, which pertains to the etiologies of bipolar disorder.

Note: The purpose is to convey just how "physical" this so-called "mental" disorder is. No need to understand it all or memorize. But get the drift—bipolar disorder is a "physical" brain illness currently miscategorized as a "mental" problem by psychiatry, with all the associated stigma and humiliation.

Bipolar Disorder and Neuroscience (Not Psychiatry!)

The following is a list of what neuroscience has uncovered, which pertains to the etiologies of bipolar disorder.

It has a strong genetic basis (genes are physical entities). Although some ingenious psychiatrist may discover "mental" genes for "mental" illnesses. As previously noted, excessive quantities of the neurotransmitter glutamate are toxic for neurons. The genes regulating glutamate transmission are GRIN1, GRIN2A, GRIN2B, GRM3, and GRM4. Genes associated with the stress response: ND4, NDUFV2, XBP1, and MTHER. For inflammation: PDE4B, IL1B, 1L6, and TNF. For apoptosis: BCC2A1 and EMPI. For oligodendrocyte-mediated myelination of white-matter tracts: CLF2B. For the Oedipus complex: BLABBER2. And of course, there are additional multiple genes relevant to bipolar disorder. Furthermore, repeated episodes of illness interfere with a process which turns genes off, termed "DNA methylation," letting the above culprit genes rev up even more. That is indeed a vicious cycle of which most psychiatrists are ignorant.

Studies of at-Risk Cohorts

These individuals have a higher likelihood of developing bipolar disorder than those in the general population. The purpose is to make an accurate diagnosis of the disease as early in its inception as possible

by research efforts to identify genetic factors, phenotypical manifestations (the set of observable traits) of an individual, which is the summation of the genes interacting with environmental variables, biomarkers, and the results of systematic imaging studies, which herald
the onset of bipolar illness." (Note: it sounds like the emperor should
be very well clothed, but in the current so-called "mental health care
system," the emperor is naked. The implications of the research find
little translation into actual psychiatric practice, which is what actual
patients experience.)

Neuroimaging in Patients with Bipolar Disorder

Two recent reviews indicated that treatment with lithium results in
increased volume in brain areas involved in mood regulation. Studies
of patients with magnetic resonance imaging (MRI) indicated that
patients who have multiple mood episodes have larger ventricles than
those with a single episode. (Note: the larger the ventricles, the greater
the demise of brain tissue—that is, neurons.)

Changes in the Ventricular Size and
Cerebral Gray Matter Volume

Those were further studies of illness course and ventricular volumes in
patients who have had multiple episodes, a single episode, or who do
not have bipolar disorder. Strakowski et al(5) utilized MRI to study
ventricular volumes in each group. Increases in volume is directly cor-
related with the number of episodes of mania. Other researchers had
similar findings.

These studies indicate that bipolar disorder is a "progressive and
deleterious disease contributing to brain tissue deterioration in the
course of recurrent episodes." The destruction of just one cubic milli-
meter of gray matter results in the death of approximately seven thousand neurons along with 10^{9th} synaptic connections, the latter nearly
equaling the number of stars in the Milky Way galaxy (approximately
200 billion!).

Brief comment: The positive findings for lithium therapy have been demonstrated, with imaging studies in bipolar disorder and significant increases in gray matter volume, yet American psychiatrists rarely prescribe it, unfortunately for their bipolar patients. Lithium requires careful medical monitoring. That is too much of a challenge for many psychiatrists in this country. Its prescription is much more commonplace in the United Kingdom, where psychiatrists are closer to being real physicians!

More on this in a bit!

Physiological Function of the Brain Networks in Bipolar Disorder

This is the connecting of different brain regions, each of which has a specific task, in which the regions share information. For example (it's not necessary to comprehend the function of each region, but to instead grasp how entire neural networks are impaired in bipolar disorder), one such network is the prefrontal-ACC-pallido-striatal-thalamus-amygdala network. Connectivity is impaired in comparison to healthy controls. A number of studies have confirmed that conclusion.

The largest difference between bipolar patients and healthy controls were seen in the connectivity between the ACC (anterior cingulate cortex) and the MIFE (medial prefrontal cortex). The latter is a critical brain region that integrates information from many other brain areas. It is intimately involved in the cognitive processes, motivation, social behavior, and the regulation of emotion.

Prefrontal Cortical Abnormalities in Bipolar Disorder

The frontal lobe is the largest of the four major lobes of the brain, the other three being the parietal, temporal, and occipital lobes. The Prefrontal Cortex (PFC) covers the front part of the frontal lobe. Its many functions enable the emergence of complex behaviors, language functions, and the capacity to make detailed plans. Through its "executive" functions, it exercises control over the limbic formations (emotional regulation and control). In a little more detail, executive functions include attentional control, cognitive inhibition, working memory, and the capacity to multitask, plan, reason, and problem-solve.

Bipolar patients, unfortunately, have reduced thickness of gray matter in the prefrontal cortex and decreased brain volume relative to healthy controls. White matter tracts demonstrate widespread abnormalities in the PFC, which negatively impacts the function of circuits and networks. One such network is the hippocampal complex: frontal lobe insula-hippocampus-thalamus and cingulate gyrus, as well as tracts to other lobes.

(Again, the names aren't important, but get the drift!) Note: the next time you want to urge a patient with bipolar disorder to "snap out of it," remember that network.

So, what are the consequences? Most psychiatrists probably don't have the slightest idea! Impaired ability to pay attention, impulsivity, inappropriate emotional responses, difficulty in interpreting the emotional meaning of facial expressions, compromised working memory, motivational difficulties, impaired ability to monitor one's behavior, and increased susceptibility to substance abuse. Above all, inadequate coping skills in the management of stress.

Imaging Differences between Bipolar and Unipolar Depression

Based on prior imaging studies, a computerized automatic algorithm has been developed utilizing the date of the differences of emotional responses to images of faces between patients with unipolar and bipolar depression. (Clinically, that differential diagnosis can sometimes be a challenge due to similarity of symptoms, even when a careful effort is made, which often does not occur in actual psychiatric practice. This is an important issue because the pharmacological treatment is different!) Note: that is a very high degree of diagnostic specificity, as good as that in internal medicine or neurology.

The computerized automated algorithm using data of emotional responses to images of faces was able to categorize unipolar and bipolar depression with 90 percent accuracy. But who is going to pay for expensive imaging studies for what psychiatry labels as "mental illness?"

Summary of Imagine Findings in Bipolar Disorder (By the Authors, Page 9)

Cumulative imaging evidence of functional, structural, and white-matter abnormalities implicates a compromised integrity of frontal-subcortical and prefrontal-limbic circuits in the pathophysiology of bipolar disorder. Additional involvement of frontal-basal ganglia-thalamic-cerebellar networks is likely. In summary, structural and functional changes support an organic basis for the emotional, cognitive, and neuroendocrine symptomatology of bipolar illness (89, 90, 199). Both regional gray-matter and white-matter changes appear to be present relatively early in disease development. Altered emotional homeostasis and cognitive difficulties stemming from these prodromal functional changes may compromise stress-coping and social adaptation, hastening the onset of bipolar illness. In some instances, there is evidence of a cumulative effect of disease duration and the number of prior episodes of brain function and structure.

Note: "An organic basis!"

Additional Research Findings in Bipolar Disorder

1. Oligodendrocyte deficiency. Also called glial cells. They provide the protective sheath (myelin) protecting the axons (main communicating projections from neurons with other neurons). There is approximately a 30 percent reduction in number.

2. Higher cortisol levels. They are associated with a 50 percent reduction of the immune system's national killer cells, which destroy cancer cells, bacteria, and viruses. The excessive levels are most likely a result of deficits in

corticolimbic regulation, amygdala over activity, and a compromised "hippocampal" regulatory role (pg. 10). Note: salivary cortisol is "elevated."

3. Circadian dysfunction. Blessed sleep. Even the close relatives of bipolar patients have less of it. Polysomnography studies of bipolar patients detect greater density of REM sleep (it is a phase of sleep characterized by rapid eye movements, a reduction in muscle tone and active dreaming, not the restful part of sleep). Sleep patterns are more variable, less efficient, with more awakenings and arousals than that of healthy individuals. Impaired sleep is associated with motivational irregularities, impaired performance, and memory function. In addition, bipolar patients have a hypersensitive melatonin response to light and a twofold greater reduction in circulating melatonin (which promotes sleep). Some "linkage" studies have associated these circadian abnormalities with genes: TIMELESS, ARNTL1, PER3, NRIDI, CLOCK, and GSK-3beta in bipolar illness (pg. 11).

4. Immune system impairment in bipolar disorder. There is a very large cast of characters. In summary, immune system dysregulation in bipolar disorder is associated with abnormal signaling of the neurotransmitter glutamate, which, in excess, injures or kills neurons. BDNF and other supportive neurotrophic factors are decreased. The result is the symptoms of the illness and serious medical comorbidities.

For those who don't mind digging a little deeper, the following detailed account of immune dysfunction in bipolar disorder does not contain a single deep emotional conflict!

Two meta-analyses (a systematic review of several studies for their quality on the same topic to reach a conclusion with greater statistical power) reported elevated levels of inflammatory cytokines (biomolecules that cause inflammation in tissue, several of which are interleukin, IL-1, T1-4, Il-6, IL-10, IL-11, IL-13, and higher level of TNK-alpha tumor necrosis factor) in bipolar patients versus non-bipolar patients. Elevated inflammation, in turn, significantly increases the risk of developing other disorders such as respiratory and gastrointestinal diseases, cardiovascular diseases, and cerebral vascular disease (examples are heart attack and stroke), as well as metabolic disorders, diabetes, dyslipidemia (elevated LDH, the bad cholesterol), and osteoporosis. Inflammatory cytokines are also found in cerebral spinal fluid (the liquid flowing around and in the brain). Imaging studies have found elevated inflammation of the subgenieal ACC, amygdala, medial PFC, basal ganglia, ventral striatum, and general nucleus accumbens, which are all real limbic components involved in the regulation of a mood and response to stress. Elevated inflammatory cytokines also suppress neurotrophic factors like BDNK and compromise the transmission of neurotransmitter anti-inflammatory cytokines. They also activate microglial cells in the brain, which, in turn, increase the inflammatory response when they start releasing reactive oxygen species, reactive nitrogen species, and more aversive cytokines. Glutamate rises to neurotoxic levels, and proapoptotic cascades are activated. Serotonin and dopamine levels in the extracellular space between synapses drops. Less efficient monoamine signaling is associated with worsening symptomatology. One study demonstrated that increased expression of inflammatory genes results in greater flow of blood in the brain, associated with emotional stimuli relative to healthy controls.

The authors summarize: "Immune dysregulation in bipolar disorder is associated with alterations of monoamine and glutamate signaling impaired neuroplasticity and neurotropic support and changes in glia) and neuronal function, most likely contributing to the symptomatic expression and medical comorbidities of this mood disorder."

One thing is truly amazing: how neuroscientific research has gleaned such detailed knowledge of the most minute physical intricacies, both normal and dysfunctional, underlying what psychiatry continues to mislabel as "mental" problems. There is a chasm between this detailed explanatory information and its practical application in the practice of the majority of psychiatrists.

Changes in Neuroplasticity and Neurotropin

Neuroplasticity is the ability of the brain to form and reorganize synaptic connections, allowing neurons to communicate. Examples are flexibility in synapse creation and adaptation, which permits learning and adopting new skills.

Alterations in GABA, GLUTAMATE AND Monoamine Transmission in Bipolar disorder

Monoamine neurotransmitter: The molecules that travel from neuron to neuron by way of synapses that make possible coordinated functions such as heart rate, breathing, sleep cycles, digestion, mood, concentration, appetite, and muscle movement. Glutamate is the chief excitatory neurotransmitter in synapses. Interestingly, it is a precursor of GABA, the brain's major inhibitory neurotransmitter. Glutamate has positive influences on learning and memory, but excessive levels are toxic to neurons.

Gamma Aminobutyric Acid (GABA): It produces a calming effect. It raises the seizure threshold. If reduces neuronal excitability and counteracts, to a degree, the excitability induced by glutamate. If glutamate dominates over GABA, neuronal integrity is undermined).

Two comprehensive meta-analyses have determined that bipolar patients have elevated levels of glutamate in the anterior cingulate cortex (ACC), medial prefrontal cortex, parieto-occipital cortex, insula, and hippocampi (pg. 15). All functionally significant brain areas compared to normal controls. This glutamatergic abnormality is consistent in all bipolar patients even when not having clinical symptoms. Aberrant glutamatergic signaling, for example, occurs in cortico-limbic regulatory pathways involved in regulating mood-state, cognitive processes, and endocrine (hormone) response. The authors state this altered glutamatergic signaling is associated with the "diverse bipolar clinical symptomatology" (pg. 15). They summarize:

"Multiple, consistent and convergent evidence from genetic, postmortem, biochemical and imaging studies, points to a principal role of glutamatergic dysregulation in the etiopathogenesis of bipolar disorder. Moreover, evidence links aberrant glial-neuron interactions and endocrine dysregulation with alteration in glutamatergic transmission" (pg. 15).

Neurotrophins are a family of proteins in the brain that promote development of proper function of neurons. They prevent apoptosis. BDNF (brain-derived neurotrophic factor) is the most studied. It is a multitasking molecule. It facilitates neural maturation, differentiation, and survival. By its involvement in nurturing synapses, it permits long-term consolidation of memories. It regulates the neurotransmitters serotonin, glutamate, and gamma-butyric acid (GABA). It promotes slow wave sleep (pg. 12). The gene for BDNF has three alleles (that means there are variant forms of the gene). Operating BDNF is actually a Dr. Jekyll and Mr. Hyde, having two basic forms, both secreted in microglia cells (which support neurons and also function as immune cells).

Pro-BDNF (PBDNF) and mature BDNF (m-BDNF): The former binds to the p7s receptor, *initiating* the shriveling of neurons and then apoptosis. M-BDNF, instead, binds to the TrkB receptor, which initiates its multiple neurotrophic actions. If you can tolerate further complexity, the three different alleles of the BDNF gene are differentiated by the substitution of methionine for valine at position 66 of the pro-domain: val66met val66val, and met66met. This BDNF gene "polymorphism" (two or more versions of a given gene) has been implicated in increased risk for developing bipolar disorder and more severe features (more clinical severity, repeated episodes, and chronicity).

There is a suggestion that suitable, competent diagnosis and pharmacotherapy elevate BDNF while reducing inflammatory mediators. In turn, that may prevent or delay progression of symptoms, encroaching disabilities, metabolic disruptions, and the progress of structural brain changes associated with debilitating apoptotic neurocognitive decline.

Changes in Intracellular Signaling Cascades

Again, this is technical. It should convey how intricate and complex are the minute physical dysregulations underlying the symptoms of bipolar disorder. It is worth a scan.

Current medications used to treat bipolar illness are of three types: the old standby, lithium, anticonvulsants like valproate, and atypical neuroleptics like aripiprazole (ability). It is likely that each, in its own fashion, has a beneficial effect on signaling cascades. The therapeutic molecules, after landing on receptors on the outer membrane of neurons, set off signaling cascades that travel through the main body of the cell, through the nuclear membrane, and ultimately to the genes. The genes respond, producing proteins that attend to a variety of cell needs and functions back in the main body. For example, the (don't sweat the big words) phospho-inosnitide-3-kinase (P13K)/AKT pathway triggers the production of growth factors, BDNF and BCL-2. Another pathway, GSK-3, regulates apoptosis, increasing activity promoting it. Downregulating GSK-3 promotes increased levels of BCL-2 and beta-catenin, which enhance cellular resilience and neuroplasticity and have antidepressant and antimanic efficiency. The three classes of medications directly and indirectly modulate the GSK-3 and P13K cascades. Also involved is the integrity of white matter in the cortico-limbic pathways critical in the regulation of mood.

Changes in Synaptic Function, Bioenergetics, and Oxidative Metabolism

(Again, don't sweat the big words). Bioenergetics refers to how organisms produce and use energy and, more specifically in this discussion, its application to neurons, supporting cells, and cell networks in the context of bipolar disorder.

The genes that code for the mitochondrial function proteins produce less than necessary for maintenance of neuroplasticity, regulation of apoptosis, maintenance of cascade signaling, and keeping the proper levels of intracellular calcium. Also, genetic deficiencies target oligodendrocyte function, which is to provide support to neurons and their axons, in particular by laying down protective coverings for axons (myelin sheath).

Telomere shortening (woe is me, as if there weren't enough "physical" abnormalities). They are to genes as aglets, the plastic or metal tips at the ends of shoelaces, are to shoelaces, serving as a protective function to prevent unraveling. If there is one thing worse than an unraveling shoelace, it's an unraveling gene. There is increased mortality due to greater vulnerability to chronic diseases. The authors hope that in reviewing immune pathologies, endocrine dysfunction, and neurotropic signaling cascades, which in turn initiate changes in gene expression that then alter the structure of the brain itself, psychiatric practice will undergo a great upgrading. They announce:

"There is a need for parallel dynamic changes in the way we diagnose and treat this condition…to significantly advance how we treat bipolar disorder." And that would rest on these newest neuroimaging, biochemical, and genetic information. There is no sign that the Diagnostic and Statistical Manual has any orientation toward the remarkably enlightening scientific information the article reviews. Research demonstrates severe mood disorders, i.e., bipolar disorder, are associated with accelerated aging, equivalent to a ten-to-fifteen-year-shorter lifespan.

The authors conclude their review of the neurobiology of bipolar disorder. Over a period of several years, rapidly advancing scientific research and findings are changing the paradigm. Instead of basing diagnosis on a description of symptomatology listed in the Psychiatric Association's Diagnostic and Statistical Manual, a more scientifically accurate basis for diagnosing and understanding the illness is beginning to emerge. Consistent findings are present at the cellular level, particularly in the interactions between neurons and glial cells. Multiple studies demonstrate the role of inflammatory processes. Vulnerability is enhanced by certain risk alleles in genes.

In summary, it should be clear bipolar disorder is not a "mental" problem but a complex "physical" disease of the brain. Psychiatry, by continuing to label it a "mental" illness and patients with the illness as "mental cases," is an obstacle to improving diagnosis and effective pharmacotherapy. Fifty percent of people affected avoid "mental health" treatment altogether, being adverse to the stigma of being labeled "mentally ill." The majority of the balance are at the mercy of an uneven, confusing, so-called "mental healthcare system" in which few therapists and the majority of psychiatrists are familiar with the details of its biological causes or the most relevant treatments of advanced "clinical psychopharmacology," which offers the most likely approach to delay and postpone debilitating brain changes that, in turn, cause debilitating symptoms, lower quality of life, and ultimately lead to serious disabilities.

What Is a Study?

When scientists and researchers wish to determine if a certain medication, particular treatment, or procedure is helpful and or harmful to a degree greater than chance, the randomized controlled trial will yield the most accurate data and answer. There are strict procedures to be followed to rule out irrelevant variables and influences that would, so to speak, contaminate the validity and reliability of a result. The subjects or patients enrolled in such a scientific study differ from one another in multiple aspects, known or unknown, which could distort the desired result or conclusion. To neutralize such variables or avoid their influencing the final answers, subjects are assigned randomly and blindly to a treatment (experimental) or control (placebo) group. Neither the patients nor the researchers have information about which patient was assigned to which group. They are "blinded." The randomized controlled trial thus will give an accurate answer about the efficacy of the treatment in relation to the nontreatment (placebo group/controlled group). Also, by means of a well-controlled clinical trial, treatments can be compared to one another.

Robert M. Post, MD

Dr. Post is a distinguished psychiatrist in the United States who, unlike the vast majority of psychiatrists in this country, decided to develop expertise in the prescription of lithium. He made the effort to become acquainted with its multiple benefits for bipolar disorder, but also for severe, recurrent unipolar depression. He spent thirty-five years of his career at the National Institute of Mental Health, and for twenty of those years, he was chief of the International Stanley Bipolar Network, aka the Bipolar Collaborative Network. He continues professional activity on behalf of lithium, emphasizing its importance to prevent the progression of the disease by reducing or preventing clinical episodes. By making a timely and accurate early diagnosis and instituting treatments that are relevant to reducing the distress of symptoms, the incapacitations which obstruct a functional and rewarding life can be minimized. The occurrence of multiple medical comorbidities and the progression to ruinous cognitive deficiencies and ultimately dementia can be delayed or prevented by effective, long-term treatment. Unlike most psychiatrists, who conceptualize severe, "recurrent" mood illness as mere "mental" problem, he realizes they can indeed result in severe brain damage unless there is sustained, targeted medical treatment.

Dr. Post comments that prescription of lithium by psychiatrists in the United States remains pathetically low in contrast to the Netherlands, Germany, and other European countries.

He reviews the work of Dr. Mogens Schou, who "was passionate about the use of lithium and compassionate about patients using lithium to better their lives."

In the preface of Dr. Schou's book, *Lithium Treatment of Mood Disorders: A Practical Guide* (April 23, 2004), it is stated:

When used correctly, lithium unquestionably produces the most dramatic benefits of any medication used to psychiatry. The aim of this practical guide is to provide patients and their families with up-to-date information about the correct use of lithium—essential knowledge they will require. A special and very important chapter deals with lithium's unique anti-suicidal effects.

When treated with lithium properly, most patients experience nothing unpleasant, but lithium has a potential to induce adverse effects. A patient who takes lithium without adequate instruction can thus run into trouble, just as a physician who is not well trained in its use.

Authorized by a renowned expert on lithium treatment, this book grew out of enormous experience and out of conviction that a well-informed patient is a critical element in effective and safe lithium treatment. In non-technical language, this guide is a complete information source for manic-depressive patients, their families and the doctors and nurses concerned with their care.

(This author would be interested in knowing how many psychiatrists in the US have actually read it, let alone implemented its treatment advice).

Source: Neuropsychopharmacology (2006) 31, 891-892, Obituary, Mogens Schou (1918-2005). He came to his interest in psychiatry and the value of lithium therapy for severe mood disorders early. His father, also a psychiatrist, was medical director of a large "mental" hospital in Denmark, and he had vivid memories of the tormented patients wandering about the wards! Electroconvulsive therapy became available in the late 1930s, and some of the severely ill patients actually recovered and could be discharged, but it then became apparent that some would relapse. Dr. Schou was keenly interested in an approach which would reduce the relapse dilemma. In 1949, he read an article by an Australian physician, John Cade, who described the benefit of lithium for manic episodes. Dr. Schou confirmed that benefit with a double-blind, placebo-controlled study. It was subsequently learned that lithium prevented recurrences of illness in bipolar and some unipolar patients. Some were critical of his work, in spite of not themselves prescribing lithium. There was a general ignorance of the long-term morbidity and mortality associated with severe mood disorders in which long-term prophylactic treatment just is not dispensed. Even though other mood-stabilizers became available, anticonvulsants and second-generation neuroleptics, he maintained that lithium has special advantages. Toward the end of his clinical practice, he was still troubled that "hidden bipolars" were not receiving lithium, "to the detriment of many patients in need. The same was true for the benefits of lithium in severe unipolar depression. Most upsetting, the documented efficacy of its effects on suicidality (reducing that often-fatal symptom by ten-fifteen times). That did not make an impression on prescribing psychiatrics, particularly in the United States, where most psychiatrists remain indifferent to this remarkable clinical benefit!

Yes, lithium is a challenging drug to use, but it can be prescribed solely by physicians who are open to prescribing it and willing to develop expertise and experience in its use. Dr. Post described the unique clinical attributes of lithium: In addition to preventing or reducing the

frequency and intensity of clinical mood episodes and de-intensify-
ing suicidal urges and impulses, it generally significantly improves the
quality of life (QOL). It reduces or eliminates cognitive damage and
the progression to dementia. Even a minute dose, 150 mg (the treatment dosage is usually 600–1,200 mg daily), in one study of elderly
women, significantly reduced the rate of cognitive deterioration versus
placebo. Another study reported a lower incidence of crimes, suicides,
and arrests in troubled adolescents. A new study from Japan demonstrated higher levels of lithium in the water supply (it is a naturally
occurring element) of certain cities was associated with lower rates of
depression and interpersonal violence in the general population compared to communities with no or lower lithium in the drinking water.

In the clinical arena, one study monitored the course of 23,712
people hospitalized for a unipolar depressive episode for seven years
after discharge. The patients who were prescribed lithium had significantly fewer rehospitalizations relative to those prescribed other medications, antidepressants, anticonvulsants, or atypical neuroleptics.

Dr. Post briefly reviews the therapeutic mechanisms of lithium,
both neuroprotective and neurotropic (processes promoting the survival of neurons). It increases the volume of the cortex and hippocampus. It increases the levels of neuroprotective proteins, BDNF
and BC1-2. It decreases other proteins like BAX and P53, which promote excessive apoptosis (hyperapoptosis). It increases neurogenesis
(the development of new neurons) and glycogenesis (which assures
the connective elements; white-matter tracts, composed of axons, are
protected through myelinization). Also supporting cells, like oligo-
dendrocytes, develop optimally and flourish. Remarkably, lithium reduces the size of lesions in other neurological disorders-hemorrhagic
stroke, traumatic brain injury, Huntington's disease, Alzheimer's disease, Parkinson's disease, amyotrophic lateral sclerosis, and other neurological lesions.

Telomeres function like aglets, which protect shoelaces from unraveling. That is a metaphor for the function of telomeres at the ends

of DNA strands. Lithium actually supports their integrity and growth, critical to health and survival. (This is how basic the actions of lithium are!) And through this action and multiple other actions, it increases longevity in humans and several animal species. It reduces all-cause mortality in severe mood illnesses.

Because lithium can impact kidney function, one must be a "real" physician to monitor it by ordering periodic renal-function tests and knowing how to "read" that data. If that is done expertly, most patients can be maintained on lithium for decades. The same is true for the thyroid gland by ordering and interpreting thyroid-function tests.

In another randomized, controlled study, the comparative efficacy of lithium was compared to an alternative mood stabilizing medication, the second-generation neuroleptic quetiapine. Multiple clinical measurements were taken. Compared with quetiapine, the outcome in those randomized to lithium was superior on all (clinical) measures, and the differences became apparent, and increasingly so, in six months of the first year.

The "Mental" Health Problem (of Psychiatry and Psychiatrists)

One would wonder why psychiatrists in the United States avoid prescribing lithium in spite of its unique properties, especially its demonstrated utility in actually reducing suicidality and special efficacy for the treatment of bipolar mood disorders. (Also, added to a regimen for severe major depression, it enhances the possibility of achieving symptom response or remission.) Well, of course, one has to prescribe and monitor lithium like a "real" physician by ordering sequential laboratory tests and interpreting the results. That alone is a challenge to many psychiatrists in the United States. It's "grubby" medicine, not at all capable of elevating their patients to a higher emotional and spiritual plane. Philosopher-doctors should not need to deal with the boringly mundane. Also, there may be an actual diagnostic entity afflicting psychiatrists. (Although they would never, ever admit it.) A phobia is defined as persistent avoidance behavior secondary to irrational fears of a specific object or activity (prescribing lithium). Please don't confront a psychiatrist with this information, however; it could lead to explosive behavior.

This aversion to prescribing lithium, however, is not entirely the fault of individual psychiatrists but also of many training programs (residencies).

Dr. Post comments in summation, "Lithium is underutilized, particularly in the United States. Many residents (psychiatrists in training) and young practitioners are not taught about the details of its use and many not be knowledgeable about some of its properties." [36]

That is a "mental" health issue on a grand scale. Who will provide the therapy to undo the lithium phobia of psychiatrists in this country? Particularly because it is their only medication that has specific anti-suicidal actions.

Schizophrenia

This is another major illness that psychiatry, in its Diagnostic and Statistical Manual, classifies as a "mental problem," although perhaps the majority do not believe patients so affected can "snap out of it," although perhaps in the public mind, many suspect, if there were a will, there would be a way.

There are an estimated 2.6 million "cases" in the United States with this "mental" problem. And most individuals with schizophrenia will become extremely symptomatic and disabled unless they are fortunate to land in the right treatment environment early in the course of the disease. You can imagine that the deep emotional conflicts are really, really deep! So deep they require ten years of deep psychiatric psychotherapy three times weekly.

Source: 1)Apoptotic mechanisms in the pathophysiology of schizophrenia, Jarskog, et al. Neuropsychopharmacology: Biological Psychiatry 2005. June 29(5) 846-58.

---

36 Principles and Practise of Psychopharmacology. Janicak, Davis, Preskorn and Ayd Jr. Lippincott, Williams Eliot Wilkins, pg. 654.

Apoptotic mechanisms in the Synaptic Pathology of Schizophrenia. Glatz, et al. Schizophrenia Research, January 2006 (81)47-65.

And if the treating psychiatrist is ignorant of dysregulated apoptosis and expert psychopharmacology to counteract it, that heavy investment in all that therapy will be a disease-extending total waste.

Even after the first episode of schizophrenia, apoptotic regulatory proteins go into overdrive. This can be so severe that there is rapid and complete elimination of nests of neurons, or, in a less severe form, nonlethal apoptosis, synapses are eliminated, though the amputated neurons may survive. This hyperapoptosis is associated with rapid clinical deterioration, intensifying symptoms, and encroaching disability. Neuroimaging studies demonstrate progressive loss of gray matter in the cerebral cortex. Gray matter contains most of the brain's neurons, which control muscles, seeing, hearing, memory, emotions, speech, decision-making and self-control—pretty much all the functions that make us human. Postmortem studies suggest a dysregulation of apoptotic proteins in several cortical areas by analyzing apoptotic regulatory proteins. This suggests intense cascades of proapoptotic proteins have led to rapid neuron death. There is also evidence of damage to DNA, its fragmentation.

This sounds quite frightening if you're the one diagnosed with schizophrenia! But in this case, it would be a blessing if the therapy-psychiatrists were right—that it's only a pathology of "deep emotional conflicts," which are resolvable in deep, deep psychoanalytically oriented psychotherapy by the brilliant use of penetrating interpretations by the psychiatrist. (Source: Progressive structural brain abnormalities and their relationship to clinical outcome: a longitudinal magnetic resonance imaging study early in schizophrenia. Beng-choon Ho, et al. Arch. Gen. Psychiatry. 2003 June 60(6): 585-94.

The course of schizophrenia is one of relatively progressive clinical deterioration, even after the first clinical episode, generally occurring in the late teens or twenties. Neuroimaging studies demonstrate progressive loss of gray and white matter. The frontal lobes are most affected, which correlates with increasing symptoms and functional impairments.

With bipolar disorder, the encroaching pathology is demonstrated by sequencing of neuroimaging studies. Cerebral spinal fluid fills spaces around the brain tissue. As the illness progresses, a greater volume of cerebral spinal fluid is inversely proportional to brain-tissue loss. Through specific analysis, the increase in cerebral spinal fluid can be carefully measured over time. In one large longitudinal MRI study at the University of Iowa, seventy-three patients were carefully determined to have schizophrenia. They were compared to twenty-three healthy control subjects. The researchers found accelerated enlargements of the cortical-sulcal spaces. (These are the typical crevices on the surface of the cortex that are filled with cerebral spinal fluid.) The gray and white matter were inversely decreased in volume. Healthy controls over the study period did not have these progressive changes. They concluded frontal lobe gray and white matter progressively declined over time, and this was associated with growing cognitive impairment of executive functions (the skills required to function independently: control of impulses, coping with problems, self-monitoring, ability to plan, ability to prioritize and complete tasks, and working memory). They also concluded that their results were consistent with other cross-sectional MRI studies of schizophrenic patients. GABA receptors in brain development function, and injury. Connie Wu and Dandan Sun. Metabolic Brain Dis. 2015 Apr. 30(2): 367-379.

GABA (gamma-aminobutyric acid) is a major neurotransmitter in the brain. What is wonderous is two things: how incomprehensively complex the brain is, as a review of this article of the GABA system makes obvious, and the majesty of the cumulative data of even this one (of multiple neurotransmitters) research has unveiled. The article is largely incomprehensible except for very specialized neuroscientists, but it highlights both points.

The following is just a superficial skim of the article. GABA is the acronym for gamma-aminobutyric acid. In the embryo brain, it sparkles in creativity, being involved in neurogenesis (the birth of new neurons). It directs neurons where to migrate, so they end up in the right location in the brain and helps them specialize and hook up to circuits. In the mature brain, in tandem with glutamate, the excitatory neurotransmitter, it maintains the inhibitory-excitatory balance necessary for proper brain function. GABA plays important roles in neurological diseases, including injury due to low oxygen (anoxic-ischemic injury), stroke, epilepsy, and traumatic brain injury. No role for GABA has yet been found for deep emotional conflicts, even though a committee of psychoanalysts is developing a theory of how GABA might be a "mental" neurotransmitter in addition to a "physical" one, although some maintain it couldn't be "physical" because they've never heard of it.

But in spite of the indifference of psychiatrists regarding GABA, researchers postulate that it plays a significant role in schizophrenia. (Which it really shouldn't, because, after all, schizophrenia is only a "mental problem.") Studies suggest the most dramatic white-matter deficit in schizophrenia links its pathology to a diminishment of the GABAergic system at both the physiological and genetic levels. White matter contains the nerve fibers (axons) that relay the messages from one neuron to other neurons. Without that communication, the brain would be as inert as a three-pound lump of clay.

And with the too-low levels of GABA, the inhibitory-excitatory balance skews toward glutamate. The further glutamate predominates, neuron dysfunction and death greatly elevate, leading to devastating diseases of the brain, Alzheimer's, amyotrophic lateral sclerosis, and Huntington's disease—but also schizophrenia? (Couldn't be, that's only a "mental problem!")

Epilepsy

Certainly, no one would debate the notion that epilepsy is a real, physical brain disease. That's just obvious from observing a person having a grand mal convulsion. In the hippocampus, normally, new neurons are born (neurogenesis), but repeated seizures are associated with rising levels of glutamate and encroaching tissue damage resulting in hippocampal sclerosis. But a similar form of hippocampal damage occurs in schizophrenia, also resulting in shrinking and damage related to runaway glutamate. Certainly "mental" glutamate does not act on the hippocampus as "physical" glutamate! Come to your senses!

Source: Anomalous brain gyrification patters in major psychiatric disorders: a systematic review and transdiagnostic integration. Sasabayash et. al. Translational Psychiatry II, Article3 number: 176 (2021).

Anomalous patterns of brain gyrification are found in major psychiatric disorders(the folds or ridges that are so apparent on the outer surface of the brain are called gyri). They are separated from one another by indentations or grooves, which are termed sulci. In the third trimester of pregnancy, gyrification occurs as the brain undergoes a considerable increase in size. The brain becomes highly convoluted, so a much greater surface area of a cortex (and therefore a great many more neurons) can fit inside the limited space of the skull (an ingenious tucking job, so to speak).

This is another long, detailed article with 161 references. The authors systematically reviewed previous magnetic resonance imaging studies of brain gyrification in schizophrenia, bipolar disorder, major depressive disorder, and autism spectrum disorder. They determined deviated gyrification patterns can differentiate patients with schizophrenia from healthy controls. This may aid in the development of biomarkers for diagnosis, rather than the current system of diagnosis, which relies only on descriptive syndromes (DSM-V). Regarding the gyral findings, the research is in a preliminary stage but may provide a new nosology informed by particular patterns of gyri: those patterns would serve as a physical indication of a given "mental" disorder, i.e., schizophrenia. (There are also other potential biomarkers for so-called "mental" disorders. Examples of biomarkers are blood pressure readings, metabolic studies (i.e., thyroid tests and others), genetic tests, or particular tissue abnormalities that are indicators of a biological factor that is identifiable for a particular disease. The authors summarize that "diverse alterations of gyrification patterns…may reflect both molecular and biochemical mechanisms. Patients with major psychiatric disorders exhibit commonly and differentially altered gyrification patterns, which suggest corresponding neural circuit changes involving the frontal and other brain regions." It is their anticipation that the development of *objective biomarkers* for the major so-called "mental" illnesses would aid in diagnosis and formulating a treatment menu based on understanding of neural circuits.

There are thirty thousand psychiatrists in the United States. It is rumored that two of them actually read the preceding article—"Schmyrification…gyrification." They concluded that it's all a bunch of phrenology! (Phrenology is a pseudoscience that held that the bumps and contours of the skull corresponded to many different character and personality traits. It fell into disrepute at the beginning of the twentieth century).

Source: Quality of life in individuals with attenuated psychiatric symptoms. The possible role of anxiety, depressive symptoms, and socio-cognitive impairments. Tackahasi, T. www.research gate.net/publication/319149566.

Attenuated psychotic symptoms are found in patients who have schizophrenia and certain other people who may not have been diagnosed with schizophrenia. The symptoms of attenuated psychotic symptoms include mild delusions, hallucinations, and disorganized speech, in the absence of a clear psychotic disorder. Some individuals with these symptoms may later progress to schizophrenia.

What is quality of life (Q.O.L.)? From *Encyclopedia Britannica*: "The degree to which an individual is healthy, comfortable, and able to participate in or enjoy life events."

This was a study of seventy-eight patients with attenuated psychotic symptoms compared to sixty-three healthy subjects. They were all assessed with interviews and specifically formulated rating scales to obtain an estimation of their day-to-day Q.O.L. Compared to healthy controls, the affected subjects had significantly lower Q.O.L. scores, with more socio-cognitive dysfunctions, anxiety, and depression. In other words, it is not fun to have a so-called "mental" illness. (One would think they would decide to "snap out of it" rather than suffer!)

Source: Mad in America, Philip Hickey, PhD.

Dr. Hickey is a retired psychologist who is an exemplar of the viewpoint that there is no such thing as "mental" illness. He has been very prolific in promoting his point of view and most likely has influenced many. He has worked in prisons (UK and US), addiction units, community mental health centers, nursing homes, and private practice. He posts on his website, "Behaviorism and Mental Health."

Source: "Alternative perspective on psychiatry's co-called mental health disorders.

(Note: this author uses the identical phrase "so-called mental illness" because that frame of reference is stigmatizing and counterproductive to preventative care at all levels, and as a large imaging literature and neuroscientific laboratory research now document, they are true (physical—not "mental" problems). They are certainly illnesses.

Hickey asserts that bipolar disorder is not an illness. He starts by laying out the DSM diagnostic criteria for bipolar disorder, the manic episode:

Manic Episode

A. A distinct period of abnormally and persistently elevated, expansive, or irritable mood and abnormally and persistently increased goal-directed activity or energy, lasting at least one week and present most of the day, nearly every day (or any duration if hospitalization is necessary).

B. During the period of mood disturbance and increased energy or activity, three (or more) of the following symptoms (four if the mood is only irritable) are present to a significant degree and representing a noticeable change from usual behavior:

1. Inflated self-esteem or grandiosity.

2. Decreased need for sleep (e.g., feels rested after only three hours of sleep).
3. More talkative than usual or pressure to keep talking.
4. Flight of ideas or subjective experience that thoughts are racing.
5. Distractibility (i.e., attention too easily drawn to unimportant or irrelevant external stimuli), as reported or observed.
6. Increase in goal-directed activity (either socially, at work or school, or sexually) or psychomotor agitation (i.e., purposeless, non-goal-directed activity).
7. Excessive involvement in activities that have a high potential for painful consequences (e.g., engaging in unrestrained buying sprees, sexual indiscretions, or foolish business investments).

C. The mood disturbance is sufficiently severe to cause marked impairment in social or occupational functioning or to necessitate hospitalization to prevent harm to self or others, or there are psychotic features.

D. The episode is not attributable to the physiological effects of substance (e.g., a drug of abuse, a medication, other treatment or to another medical condition.

Note: A full manic episode that emerges during antidepressant treatment (e.g., medication, electroconvulsive therapy) but persists at a fully syndromal level beyond the physiological effect of that treatment is sufficient evidence for a manic episode and, therefore, a Bipolar I diagnosis.

Note: Criteria A-D constitute a manic episode. At least one lifetime manic episode is required for the diagnosis of Bipolar I disorder.

He comments on criterion A that the very basis for the diagnosis of bipolar disorder "is either feeling particularly good about everything or feeling particularly grumpy and angry." He observes that it's not logical for an illness to manifest itself in such diametrically opposite states: "This is indeed a strange illness." He turns to criterion B: at least three symptoms listed must be present to make the diagnosis. He questions why three symptoms…why not two or four? He notes how different the clinical picture would be if the patient has symptoms one, three, and four versus two, five, and seven. "The notion that these two presentations are in fact manifestations of the same illness is untenable" and exists solely because the APA (American Psychiatric Association) mandated it. He next reviews each symptom.

1. Inflated self-esteem or grandiosity. He notes that making a judgment about this symptom on the part of a mental health care professional is "intrinsically subjective and unreliable."
2. Decreased need for sleep. He notes many individuals manage quite well on four or five hours sleep.
3. More talkative than usual or pressure to keep talking. He notes some adults carry this trait from childhood, and it is a result of poor training during childhood for those who talk excessively.
4. Flight of ideas or the subjective experience that thoughts are racing. He notes, "Most people experience flight of ideas on a fairly regular basis…it's called stream of consciousness, and it flows like a babbling brook." It also is a product of deficient parental discipline in childhood.
5. Distractibility (i.e., attention easily drawn to unimportant or irrelevant external stimuli). He notes that this "is the same thing as the flight of ideas" and adds, "so you get two hits for the price of one. The primary purpose of the DSM is to generate business for psychiatrists."
6. Increase in goal-directed activity (either socially, at work or school, or sexually), or psychomotor agitation. He states,

"the real issue here is not goal-directed activity as such, but rather, irresponsible and inconsiderate activity." Traits of responsibility and consideration for others, if not instilled in childhood through parental discipline, will manifest in adulthood as irresponsibility (i.e., you're not ill; you're bad).

7. Excessive involvement in pleasurable activities that have a high potential for painful consequences (e.g., engaging in unrestrained buying sprees, sexual indiscretions, or foolish business investments). He comments, "Once again, what is involved here is what most people would call irresponsibility." Such "self-indulgent" behavior is present is a function of earlier upbringing and not due to a disease "like diabetes...best treated with drugs."

He also comments on lithium (a primary mood-stabilizer prescribed in bipolar disorder: it has a "calming effect" on all individuals, as does beer. "A couple of beers can be very effective in helping shy people overcome their inhibitions. Very few rational people would conclude from this that shyness is an illness and alcohol a "medication." Just as a shy person can face their shyness and change, so "the manically irresponsible person can acknowledge his problem behaviors and tackle them in a normal way." If such a patient does take lithium, he needs to be aware, or like alcohol, it also has some long-term side effects.

He rounds out his discussion by saying, "The so-called mental illnesses are problems that do *not* require medical help." The American Psychiatric Association is the psychiatrists' trade union," which has been enormously successful in classifying human problems into mental illnesses, which legitimates their prescribing practices for the purpose of making a very comfortable income." He objects to "the spurious notions that these pharmaceutical products are medicines, and that they are being prescribed to combat illnesses."

Note: Dr. Philip Hickey's website, as of January 1, 2022, is accessible to the general public. For a symptomatic person, perhaps confused and in a muddle about his dysphorias and where to turn for some relief, how will he be impacted by Dr. Hickey's material? Dr. Hickey has very pronounced acerbic commentary about psychiatry, but psychiatry is as indifferent as ever to the medical model; the exalted philosopher sages that they cannot deign to robustly respond to Dr. Hickey's gross distortions, leaving their "mental cases" dangling in uncertainty (particularly if they are influenced by Dr. Hickey's paradigm).

Source: "How Psychiatry Turned General Difficulties in Adaptation into "Real Illnesses Just like Diabetes," Philip Hickey, Ph.D. http://www.behaviorism and mental health.com

Of course, people can have "difficulties in adaptation" to which they react with symptoms, depression, anxieties, guilt, distractibility, behavioral problems, etc., as understandable, responsible responses to a wide variety of stresses. But over the past century, and particularly since the discovery of "psychotropic" drugs, psychiatry has constructed a huge variety of what they categorize as "mental" illnesses that need to be treated with drugs, so they pronounce that such illnesses, which they also term "diseases," warrant those terms because they result in functional difficulties and impairments. There is no reference to associated physical or biological abnormalities, which, in all other medical specialties, are an integral element in diagnosable disease. In other words, there must be an identifiable biological etiology or cause. In psychiatry's case, there would need to be an identifiable physical abnormality of the brain if any condition were to be categorized as a disease.

Yet the absence of demonstrable physical etiologies for their so-called "mental" illnesses was overcome by their assertion that the sine qua non for identifying the presence of a disease is the dysfunction associated with a given symptomatic picture. Hence the birth of the Diagnostic and Statistical of Manual of "Mental" Disorders (this author placed the quotes on "Mental").

The DSM thus promotes psychosis, psychoneurosis, and personality disorders under the disease rubric.

The mode of classifying mental symptoms into mental illnesses got an added impetus with the advent of psychotropic drugs. "It was all the more critical to convince the public, the media, the rank-and-file psychiatrists and real doctors that psychiatric disorders were in fact real illnesses, just like diabetes." Psychiatry also learned to present mental illnesses as actually having a physical basis—that is, the so-called "imbalance" of neurotransmitters. They have held on to that explanation even though there has never been any actual scientific proof of it. Dr. Hickey summarizes, "It turned out to be one of the biggest lies in the history of medical science."

Next, a collaboration was established. Big Pharma continued to manufacture an ever-expanding list of so-called psychotropics, and of course, that required an ever-expanding network of psychiatrists to prescribe them. And of course, the pharmaceutical industry has deep pockets, showering them with sumptuous meals at the finest restaurants and even weekend trips to luxury hotels in popular tourist locations. This joint venture, Big Pharma and psychiatry, was highly successful. Some of the biggest-selling drugs in all of medicine are psychotropics, i.e., Prozac and Zoloft, to say nothing of Aripiprazole (Abilify), a second-generation neuroleptic.

Dr. Hickey refers to "Taber's Cyclopedic Medical Dictionary" (edition 22), which explains the biological abnormalities which cause all diseases (actual illnesses). Tuberculosis is an infectious disease caused by the tubercle bacillus, Mycobacterium tuberculosis. Pneumonia is an inflammation of the lungs due to an infection by a pathogen. Myocardial infarction is a disease of the heart in which living heart muscle dies due to anoxia secondary to an occlusion of a coronary artery, etc. This very basic relationship of real disease to particular biological abnormalities is, of course, absent for the so-called "mental" illnesses.

He states that to determine the level of impairment, "one needs to demonstrate the characteristic pathology, and that requires laboratory and imaging techniques before a definitive diagnosis can be made. In the absence of those, psychiatric diagnoses are not describing actual diseases. This is psychiatry's most profound sense of embarrassment. They gambled their entire professional standing on the belief of the famous theory of chemical imbalance would be proven…it hasn't been." He continues, "Intellectually, and conceptually, psychiatry is dead. The corpse, however, continues to be supported by the pharmaceutical industry, although that cannot last forever. Gradually, psychiatry will slip quietly and ignominiously into the morass of scientific wrong turns, iatrogenic damage, and oral degeneracy."

Source: Speak Out Against Electric Shocks. Philip Hickey, PhD. January 15, 2018.

When Dr. Hickey speaks about "high-voltage electric shocks," he is apparently referring to a rather older form of treatment for severe major depressive disorder, electroconvulsive therapy (ECT), first used in the 1930s in Italy.

He gives examples of the plight of two individuals after they had a course of ECT. Helen Crane was treated in the late 1990s. She blamed the treatments for wiping out years of her memories of trips abroad for dramatic family events. She had forgotten her mother had passed away. "It was devastating going through bereavement again." Deborah Schwartzkopff had sixty-six ECT treatments over the course of three years. There were such "gaping holes in her memory" that she couldn't recall her wedding or the birth of her children. Her marriage of twenty-eight years ended. "I couldn't remember my relationship, and without those memories, I had no emotional connection," she said. There are numerous complaints and warnings about ECT in the media and by professionals. "Critics of ECT claim around a third of patients will notice some sort of permanent change from problems with speech and basic skills like addition." The treatment "doesn't last, and three or four weeks later, the person is either back at the same level of depression or, many studies show, worse levels of depression." Dr. Hickey quotes from the informational brochure on ECT from Mt. Sinai Hospital in

New York City, in which it states, "As with any medical procedure, ECT carries its own set of risks, which need to be balanced against its benefits…ECT is one of the safest procedures performed under general anesthesia." Dr. Hickey comments that there "is no mention of permanent loss of pre-shock memories or the devastating effects that this can entail." The approach the psychiatrists take is the "total suppression of information concerning the harmful, extensive, and often permanent effects of *high voltage electric shocks* to the brain." He quotes a British psychiatrist, author of *The Myth of the Chemical Cure*, which also critiques "electric shocks."

"A few weeks after the ECT has taken place, people are no better than they would have been if they had never had it."

ECT also results in "cognitive impairment, disorientation, impaired attention and memory." In addition, it results in "a state of disturbed behavior similar to mania and sometimes with frank psychotic features." Peter Breggin describes such side effects of ECT as being "reminiscent of other brain diseases such as the late stage of multiple sclerosis." The late neurologist John Friedberg, MD, reviewed the neuropathology resulting from ECT in experimental animals and humans, which include "petechial hemorrhage, gliosis, and neuronal loss." He concluded that ECT results in brain disease, and he "questions whether doctors should offer brain damage to their patients."

In summary, Dr. Hickey states: "There are truly no depths of deception and spin to which psychiatrists will not go to promote the fiction that they are real doctors, treating real illnesses with bona fide, safe, and effective treatments. In reality, psychiatry is a self-serving, destructive, disempowering, and stigmatizing hoax, which, like all hoaxes, fears nothing more than exposure. We need to keep exposing this hoax, especially including firsthand accounts from people who have been hurt by psychiatry, whose voices have been suppressed for far too long.

"Calling for the suppression of those voices, on the pretense that they promote *bias*, is just another example of psychiatric arrogance.

How dare you challenge us; we're real doctors, you know, and we have white coats and shock machines to prove it. You're just a patient.

"Psychiatry is utterly and totally irredeemable. It simply needs to go away."

One wonders how many "hits" there have been on Dr. Hickey's website. At least 50 percent of people with the symptoms of so-called "mental" illnesses never seek help at all in the so-called "mental health care system." He and his fellow travelers play a role in this.

An important note of clarification: Dr. Hickey does not believe there are actual "mental" illnesses and all "mental symptoms are explainable as understandable responses to stresses, difficult circumstances, and trauma, so in that sense, he could logically use the term "so-called mental illness." This author uses the same terminology not because he doesn't believe that they aren't genuine disease-entities but because evidence should dictate that the whole "mental" frame of reference is misleading and stigmatizing. They are "physical," *not* "mental," diseases.

Psychiatric Drugs

Those who are suffering and who come across Dr. Hickey's website will absorb a very negative assessment of the drugs psychiatrists prescribe. They are presented as being a product of a collaboration between pharmaceutical companies and psychiatrists, used not to benefit patients but to build profits for the pharmaceutical companies and legitimize the practices of psychiatrists, who can then write prescriptions like physicians in other medical specialties, allowing them the pretense they too are "real" doctors. The psychiatric drugs are relegated to a particular category of offensiveness, giving the impression they are never therapeutic and uniquely result in adverse circumstances. It is not an appetizing portrayal of these drugs.

Source: The FDA: Drug Review Process: Ensuring Drugs are Safe and Effective. (http://www.fda.gov/drugs/information.)

The FDA does not discriminate. It is an equal-opportunity employer, so to speak. It does not assign the drugs the psychiatrists prescribe to a lower level of assessment for safety and efficacy. All drugs prescribed in the United States undergo the same scrutiny.

The path a drug travels from a lab to your medicine cabinet is usually long. A brief synopsis: Drugs must first undergo preclinical (animal) testing before the FDA initiates a "rigorous evaluation process which scrutinizes everything about the drug." The FDA, after reviewing relevant data, then decides "whether it is reasonably safe for the company (the drug developer) to move forward with testing the drug in humans." Before clinical trials can begin, all relevant data is also reviewed by an independent panel of scientists and nonscientists in hospitals and research institutions. They also decide on the safety of the protocols for the proposed clinical studies.

Phase I studies are usually conducted on healthy volunteers. Phase II studies begin if those I studies don't find evidence of toxicity. These are controlled trials in which patients receiving the drug being evaluated are compared to a similar number of patients receiving an inactive substance (placebo). Phase III studies are then planned if the results of Phase II show evidence of efficacy and safety. These are the very large, double-blind randomized trials employing up to three thousand patients. These studies "gather more information about safety and effectiveness." Finally, the drug's sponsor must submit to the FDA a New Drug Application (NDA) before the FDA makes a final determination.

"This is the formal step a drug sponsor takes to ask the FDA to consider approving a new drug for marketing in the United States."

Why do American psychiatrists avoid prescribing lithium for bipolar disorder? It's as if bipolar disorder and lithium are meant to marry. This simple salt is a multitasker in the brain of bipolar patients. So many of its varied therapeutic actions speak to the multiple physical dysregulations, the pathophysiologies of the disease. Yet it is the most under-prescribed medication for psychiatric patients. It's as if internists refused to write prescriptions for statin drugs to treat cholesterol because sometimes serious side effects occur. Prescribing lithium requires the prescriber to function like a *real physician*, weighing risks versus benefits, watching for contraindications and drug interactions, ordering and monitoring laboratory tests, monitoring for side effects, avoiding toxicity, and measuring benefits. That's just too much of a challenge for the average psychiatrist. Besides, it's a grubby business compared to lifting the patient into new epiphanies of emotional advancement in deep psycho-analytic psychotherapy.

Source: World Psychiatry: "Lithium vs. valproate vs. olanzapine vs. quetiapine as maintenance monotherapy for bipolar disorder…" Joseph F. Hayes et. al. 01 February 2016.

This study was conducted to determine which maintenance treatment for bipolar disorder is superior in clinical practice. They compared four medications, lithium, valproate (an anticonvulsant), olanzapine (an atypical neuroleptic), and quetiapine (another atypical neuroleptic) in what is called a "population-based cohort study." The medical records of 5,089 patients with bipolar disorder were reviewed with the objective of determining which of four medications used as monotherapy (that is, the drug is used by itself, with no other drug added) to determine which medication maintained a remission of symptoms the longest (the duration of successful monotherapy). The four medications: lithium (N-505 patients), valproate (N-1173), olanzapine (N-1366), and quetiapine (N-1075). Treatment failure was defined as time to stopping medication due to adverse effects, or time to needing an additional medication added due to symptomatic worsening. (In the pharmacotherapy of bipolar disorder, usually two or more medications are required.) The duration of successful monotherapy was significantly longer with lithium (2.05 years) compared with .76 years for quetiapine, .98 years for valproate, and 1.03 years for olanzapine. The authors summarized:

"Lithium appears to be more successful as monotherapy maintenance treatment than valproate, olanzapine, or quetiapine."

Note: starting treatment with one of the other drugs will shorten the time in which another drug will have to be added, increasing the risk of adverse effects due to polypharmacy (the prescribing of two or more medications for a given purpose).

And there will be more to say about lithium because severe, extreme clinical depression is a precipitant of suicidality, and lithium is the only known medication which reduces suicidality significantly.

And yet American psychiatrists refuse to prescribe it! They just don't want to. They just don't know how! Instead, they use one of the other medications, which do not have the same degree of anti-suicidal benefit!

Psychiatry should not be considered a medical specialty until every psychiatrist expertly prescribes lithium. It is their patients who are unnecessarily dying, not them!

Source: "Lithium Top Treatment for Prevention of Bipolar Disorder Rehospitalization," b.p. Magazine, 6 Aug. 2018. This article summarized the results of a study completed at the Karolinska Institute in Sweden and published in *JAMA Psychiatry*. The researchers studied the readmission rate of eighteen thousand Finish patients who had previous admissions for bipolar disorder. They were followed in the study over seven years. Patients treated with lithium had a 30 percent lower readmission rate. The most commonly prescribed neuroleptic (atypical antipsychotic) used to treat bipolar disorder, by contrast, had only a 7 percent reduction. The researchers concluded that lithium is the most effective option to treat bipolar disorder and that it should be the first line of treatment. Second-best was injections of long-acting neuroleptics.

It's possible that American psychiatrists enjoy admitting bipolar patients into hospitals, and that's why they don't prescribe lithium.

Source: "An Oldie But Goodie: Lithium in the Treatment of Bipolar Disorder through neuroprotective and Neurotropic Mechanisms." International Journal of Molecular Sciences. Eunsoo Won and Yong-ku Kim, 11 December 2017.

Neuroprotection refers to the ability of a treatment to prevent neurons from being degraded and ultimately dying. Neurotropism refers to processes that facilitate neuronal robustness and survival as well as the development of new neurons from neural stem cells. The authors summarize modern studies with reliable designs and updated guidelines, which recommend that lithium should be the treatment of choice for bipolar disorder in all of the disease's four phases, acute manic episodes, mixed episodes, depressive episodes, and long-term prophylaxis. They review some of lithium's specific therapeutic mechanisms in the treatment of the disease (don't worry about the definitions—just note the reality of the physicality of the disease's pathophysiology): it directly inhibits glycogen synthase kinase 3B and regulates neurotrophic factors, neurotransmitters, oxidative metabolism, apoptosis, second messenger systems, and other *biological* (emphasis mine) systems. Ultimately, it is associated with neuronal plasticity (the ability of neurons and neural networks to adaptively change activity, in response to intrinsic or external demands, by reorganizing its structure, functions, or connections).

If any psychiatrist, by chance, should read this article, it contains a complete "how-to" for the prescription of this therapeutic molecule, which gives so much to so few (in the United States!).

Source: Challenging the Negative Perception of Lithium and Optimizing its Long-term Administration. Janusz K. Rybakowski. Department of Adult Psychiatry, Poznan University of Medical Sciences, Poznan, Poland.

Even this distinguished psychiatrist in Poland is distressed by *how little* American psychiatrists prescribe lithium.

Dr. Janus K. Rybakowski of Poznan University has been a lithium expert for decades. "Despite such hard evidence for efficacy and favorable effects of the administration of lithium in bipolar illness, it is greatly underutilized."

In particular, he "*deplores*" that it is even more underutilized in the United States than in Europe, in spite of its "multiple assets." He reviews the extensive research that establishes its efficacy, multiple placebo-controlled studies over decades. In the twenty-first century, lithium's prophylactic efficacy "was abundantly demonstrated" in three meta-analyses. (A meta-analysis is a statistical analysis that combines the results of several well-performed scientific studies to derive the most accurate possible result or conclusion. Lithium has had an undeserved reputation as a "toxic" drug, most likely because American psychiatrists who prescribed it decades ago were incompetent in its prescription.)

He reviews lithium's multiple assets for the treatment of bipolar disorder, its antidepressant action, its suicide prevention properties, its pro-cognitive and anti-dementia effects, as well as the reduced frequency of other debilitating medical illnesses. He comments that potential serious side effects, kidney or thyroid issues, can be managed by a psychiatrist who bothers to practice like a real physician (this author's opinion) and is also willing to absorb some knowledge of kidney function (nephrology). He discusses in detail how to manage those issues, guided by safety concerns and practices.

And there is a significant percentage of bipolar patients who have an excellent response to lithium. (If it is rarely prescribed by psychiatrists in the United States, these patients will never be identified. So, they are allowed to suffer and deteriorate on less optimal mood stabilizers.)

About a third to a quarter of bipolar patients will do very well on long-term monotherapy with lithium, according to Dr. Rybakowski. These patients experienced "a dramatic change in their lives as their mood episodes were prevented." They researched sixty patients who had been placed on lithium prophylaxis in the 1970s and forty-nine more, from the 1980s, who had been monitored on lithium long-term. A decrease in the neurotropic protein BDNF in serum is a marker of later-stage illness. In these patients, however, BDNF levels were normal, equal to those of healthy controls even over the passage of decades. These fortunate responders did not experience the clinical, neurobiological, or neurocognitive manifestations of the progression of the disease in the brain. The concentrations of neurotoxic cytokines were in the normal range. They also described five patients who were lithium long-termers (two men and three women), who had been maintained on lithium for over forty years. There was no progression of the disease. They had all been started early after the onset of symptoms. They had maintained normal cognitive and professional activity as well as optimal functioning in family and social roles. His team concluded, "Patients with a favorable response to lithium such longitudinal administration of lithium can produce satisfactory performance in vocational and psychosocial areas…and the management of potential adverse effects can be adequate."

Dr. Rybakowski concluded that lithium should be started after the first episode of bipolar disorder because of its favorable influence on the neuro-progression of the illness."

Electroconvulsive Therapy
("High-voltage electric shocks"—Dr. Hickey)

Source: "Electroconvulsive Therapy: A History of the Controversy, but Also of Help." Jonathan Sadowsky, PhD., January 13, 2017, Scientific American.

But first, this author's brief comments: it should be a cause for major scandal. It is hard to believe, but "high-voltage electric shocks" are still being given at the Mayo Clinic, Tufts Medical Center, Beth Israel Deaconess Medical Center, McLean Hospital, and Massachusetts General Hospital (Harvard). Obviously, the physicians and administrators who have authorized this procedure to be performed in their facilities have not gotten the latest scientific information about the procedure from Dr. Philip Hickey, PhD.

The author of this article, Dr. Sadowsky, was struck by a discrepancy. Critics portray ECT as a form of medical abuse, yet some psychiatrists and, more importantly, patients consider it to be safe and effective. Few medical treatments have such disparate images.

Dr. Sadowsky is a historian of psychiatry at Case Western Reserve University. He published a book on the history of ECT (electroconvulsive therapy). He was interested in learning, "Why has this treatment been so controversial?" Of course, it sounds painful, inducing seizures with a direct electric stimulus, but that doesn't explain the controversy, as other medical treatments—for example, chemotherapy for cancer—produce physical distress. Psychiatrists in the 1930s discovered that the induction of seizures relieved some patients with severe "mental" illness of the worst of their symptoms. Seizures were induced with the use of a chemical, Metrazol. Unfortunately, before the onset of the seizure, patients experienced an interval of extreme terror, which they remembered after the seizure. Italian researchers, who developed ECT, had done so with the objective of making seizure induction "more humane and less fearsome." Their new method was rapidly adopted in most countries. Unfortunately, to an uninformed observer, ECT still looked barbaric, as patients would have full-blown convulsions, though under controlled circumstances. Such was portrayed in the film *One Flew over the Cuckoo's Nest*, in which an unruly patient is subjected to the procedure as a punishment. Even though the movie was released in 1975, it depicted a period of the 1950s when, indeed, the procedure looked primitive. The author explains that since then, the procedure has been refined. The patient is given anesthesia first, then a muscle relaxant. The seizure is highly modified, visible generally only in the big toes. After the procedure, in the recovery room, when they awaken, they are not uncomfortable.

So, one source of the controversy was the image of the unmodified treatment itself, and perhaps its misuse in some unethical facilities in its earliest days. Even though, by the 1960s, the evidence that ECT was very effective for treating depression was scientifically credible, there entered on the scene the "anti-psychiatry movement," which rejected the very idea of mental illness, physical treatments, and especially ECT. It aroused their strongest protestations. The author notes, however, that more recently, "There have been a growing number of positive portrayals," often in patient memoirs like Carrie Fisher's, Norman Mailer's, and Martha Manning's, "of how ECT brought them back from bleak depression." Perhaps "the main source of controversy concerns a possible adverse effect: memory loss, but "many patients say they have little if any memory loss." Although permanent, long-term memory loss can be an adverse effect, "many clinicians believe it to be exceedingly rare, based on their experience treating many patients over the years."

This author's note: ECT is generally not given on a daily basis. The competent psychiatrist should evaluate the patient the day after each treatment as to symptoms and memory status. The key to avoiding severe memory disruption is to be attentive to the patient's status after each treatment! This is most likely done at the medical centers previously mentioned. (Note: It is possible that at a few facilities with low standards, a psychiatrist will order a series of six to ten treatments without seriously evaluating the patient on a serial basis. If so, that would explain unnecessary memory impairment.)

This author's experience with some patients who benefitted from a course of ECT (of course, none of the patients had a "real" illness, as per Dr. Hickey), and so what kind of malevolence is involved in subjecting them to "high-voltage electric shocks?"

Severe major depression presents in different ways. A gentleman, a WWII veteran, was hospitalized with a total breakdown. He had survived the war in Europe and had a reasonably successful life. As a senior, he had an infection in a limb, which was soon followed by a "nervous breakdown." When evaluated, he just stared ahead. He could not respond verbally to questions during the evaluation. He was mute. He didn't follow directions. He was sweating. Slowly, after three or four ECT treatments, he began to respond. He had been through a nightmare, which took him quite a while to even begin to understand.

A lovely, middle-aged woman was evaluated in the hospital. Her husband was in attendance. But she was not lovely during the evaluation. She was guarded and suspicious, with an underlying hostility. Her husband clarified that she had had one or two similar episodes previously. She was engrossed in fearful delusions of her life being in jeopardy from a sinister organization. She could not rest. But that was not her! In reality, after her third or fourth treatment, she became gracious and charming. She was an accomplished artist. Her husband, equally charming, was a connoisseur of roses.

Another middle-aged woman was in the hospital. She was obviously grossly agitated. She couldn't stop pacing and wringing her hands. Her facial expression was distorted by distress. Finally, after a few ECT treatments, she became much calmer and peaceful. She could hold a conversation.

Another middle-aged woman was just immobile. When taken to the ECT suite, she just lay flat, as if she were devoid of muscle tone. She did not communicate, having a vacant stare. After several ECT treatments, a person started to emerge.

But none of these people had an illness per Dr. Hickey, and there was no reason to subject them to "high-voltage electric shocks!"

Mental Symptoms (Come On, Just Pull Yourself up by Your Bootstraps!)

One prominent habit of the so-called anti-psychiatry coalition, e.g., Dr. Philip Hickey is a card-carrying member, is the strict classification of illness as either "physical" or "mental" (not that organized psychiatry doesn't do the same). Physical illnesses are said to have distinctive biological abnormalities that can be demonstratable through biologically based imaging or laboratory studies. "Mental" illnesses, however, are said to lack a physical pathological basis and therefore are not truly real illnesses. (Psychiatry does not go that far, as Dr. Hickey points out. Psychiatry moves the goalposts by nullifying the requirement there must be some underlying physical pathology by instead invoking "functional" impairment as the sine qua non for defining symptoms that constitute illness or disease. According to Dr. Hickey, unless a pathological lesion is present, symptoms are merely *understandable* emotional reactions to stressful or difficult circumstances.

But there is a question Dr. Hickey ignores or is ignorant of: "real" physical illnesses, in many contexts, produce (unreal?) "mental" symptoms and often come to the attention of health care providers by dint of the "mental" symptoms. (Could it be that the "mental" symptoms are merely a normal, understandable reaction to having a "real" physical disease?)

Note: Unfortunately, the author of this article, written in 2002, a psychiatrist, Ronald J. Diamond, MD, adheres to the antiquated notion that so-called "mental" illnesses are "psychological" problems. In contrast to physical illnesses...The "psychological" problem of depression can arise from abnormally low thyroid hormone. The "psychological" problem of panic attacks can be caused by epinephrine secreting tumors (pheochromocytomas), marked by abnormal personality changes, characterized aggressiveness, and marital conflict, or can be caused by brain tumors. He lists a series of studies that document people with "mental" symptoms often have underlying "physical" illness, which causes the "mental" symptoms.

A 1989 study by Sax et al. evaluated 509 patients at community mental health centers. At least 39 percent "had at least one active important physical disease" (but not the majority). He goes on, "The question is, what medical illness can cause depression, anxiety, etc.? The problem is that depression, caused by a brain tumor, may be identical to depression caused by marital discord or endogenous depression." He comments on the fact that "a huge number of illnesses can present as depression, and the vast majority of these illnesses can also present as anxiety or delirium."

Next, he undertakes the task of trying to organize illnesses by their "psychological" effects. He starts by noting that "there is a tendency to assume that all psychiatric patients are just 'nuts,' without real illness, on the part of many physicians." But the "mental" symptoms may be a mask: hysterical symptoms may originate in patients with multiple sclerosis, irrationally from a slow bleed inside the skull due to a subdural hematoma. Depression in association with unusual dryness of the skin and complaints of feeling cold can occur in hypothyroidism.

There is a long list of illnesses that can present with psychotic symptoms, for example, neurological illnesses, (multiple sclerosis, Huntington's chorea, Pick's disease, encephalitis, HIV, brain abscess) and metabolic disorders (severe liver and kidney disease, electrolyte disturbances, acute intermittent porphyria, Wilson disease, etc.).

There are other categories, each with subcategories of specific diseases that present with "mental" symptoms. So, this long list of "physical" illnesses is often linked with "mental" symptoms such as psychosis.

The symptomatic expressions of depression and anxiety are associated with equally long lists of physical diseases. Their so-called "mental" symptoms are apparently intimately linked to physical diseases and should not be separated from them, isolated from them, as if they're categorically totally different.

Psychiatric Diagnosis: Everyone Is an "Expert" When It Comes to "Mental" Illnesses

Source: Science Daily, July 8, 2019. "Psychiatric Diagnosis Is Scientifically Meaningless."

This was a synopsis from the journal *Psychiatry Research* of a study from the University of Liverpool that concluded "that psychiatric diagnoses are worthless as tools to identify discrete mental health disorders." The Liverpool research focused on five diagnostic entities directly from the DSM-5: schizophrenia, bipolar disorder, depressive disorders, anxiety disorders, and trauma-related disorders. Their main conclusions were that there was high overlap of symptoms between diagnoses and that they gave little useful information about individual patients or what treatment might be beneficial. The lead researcher, Dr. Kate Alsopp of the University of Liverpool, is quoted:

"Although diagnostic labels create the illusion of an explanation, they are scientifically meaningless and can create stigma and prejudice. I hope these findings will encourage mental health professional to think beyond diagnoses and consider other explanations of mental distress, such as trauma and other adverse life experiences."

And Professor Peter Kinderman from the University of Liverpool said:

"This study provides yet more evidence that the bio-medical diagnostic approach in psychiatry is not fit for purpose. Diagnoses frequently and uncritically reported as "real illnesses" are in fact made on the basis of internally inconsistent, confused, and contradictory patterns of largely arbitrary criteria. The diagnostic system wrongly assumes that all distress results from disorder and relies heavily on subjective judgments about what is normal."

(Note: the researchers at the University of East London may have overreached. No matter how they are classified, these are disease entities that cause severe symptoms, suffering, disabilities and premature death.)

Professor John Read of the University of East London said: "Perhaps it is time we stopped pretending that medical-sounding labels contribute anything to our understanding of the complex causes of human distress or of what kind of help we need when distressed."

The original article from which *Scientific Daily* extrapolated was: Kate Allsopp, John Read, Rhiannon Corcoran, Peter Kinderman. Heterogenally in psychiatric diagnostic classification. *Psychiatric Research*, 2019; 279: 15 DOI: 10, 1016/j.psychres.2019.07.005

This author thanks *Scientific Daily* for making the original article more intelligible, as it was somewhat abstruse.

The Meanings of Madness. Bookshelf by Stephen Eide. A review of DSM: A History of Psychiatry's Bible by Allan V. Horwitz, Johns Hopkins.

This is a book report. According to the report's author, Stephen Eide, Professor Allan Horwitz, a sociologist at Rutgers University, critiques the DSM-5 and makes two main points about it. The first is that it's a "social creation," the second that "we're stuck with it." The DSM made its first appearance in 1952, and by 1980, it was in wide use. Its diagnostic codes, in a similar fashion to codes for medical illnesses, are used by providers and insurance companies to facilitate payments for services. Mr. Horwitz believes, in spite of the abundance of codes—approximately three hundred—they don't identify actual legitimate mental disorders. "Diagnostic criteria must portray evidence-based empirical research," but the DSM-5 codes "emerge from uncertainty factionalism and intense political conflicts, economic considerations, and other interests." But he does acknowledge the DSM-5 serves a legitimate societal purpose. "In the past, undermining psychiatry has tended to make worse off these Americans who, without question, suffer from incapacitating psychiatric disorders. Somewhere around 500,000 severely mentally ill people are either institutionalized, incarcerated, or homeless. Unless we're going to tell such vulnerable people 'to snap out of it' and get a job, psychiatry has a place in American society."

Research Domain Criteria

In 2008, at the US National Institute of Mental Health (NIM), it was decided to create a new approach to diagnosis in psychiatry. The DSM, having only a symptom-based approach, was considered deficient, since it does not integrate the newer genetic imaging studies and neuroscience findings, thus limiting possible scientific progress. The new plan in development is intended to link the basic biological and behavioral components with the objective of refining the capacity to elucidate more basic causes and develop more targeted treatments. Dr. Insel, the director, discussed the rationale: "Patients with mental disorders deserve better...I look at the data, and I'm concerned...I don't see a reduction in the rate of suicide or prevalence of mental illness or any measure of morbidity. I see it in other areas of medicine, and I don't see it for mental illness. That was the basis for my comment that people with mental illness deserve better."

(This author's note: even a new diagnostic system would fail to result in the improvements the good doctor desires because of the structural deformities of the current "mental health care system," racked by stigma and gaping holes in efficiency. An example, for the symptoms, its construct: "Acute Threat." (fear)

Negative Valence Systems, as of January 2022

Construct/ Subconstruct	Molecules	Cells	Neural Circuits
Acute Threat ("Fear")	BDNF * CCK * Cortisol / Corticosterone * CRF family * Dopamine * Endogenous cannabinoid * FGF2 * GABA * Glutamate * Neuropeptide S * Neurosteroid* NMDAR * NPY * OX * Oxytocin * Serotonin * Vasopressin	BABAergic cells * Glia * Neuron * Pyramidal cell	Amygdala (basal * AceN * lateral * medial) * ACC (dorsal * rostral) * Autonomic nervous system * Hippocampus (posterior * anterior) * Hypothalamus * ICMs * Insular cortex * OFC * PAG (dPAG * vPAG) * Pons (LC) * PFC (vmPFC (ll) * dmPFC (pl) * LOPFC/ insula * RPVM
Physiology	Behavior (Symptoms)	Self-reports	Paradigms
BP * EDA * EMG (facial) * Eye tracking * Heart rater * Pupillometry * Breathing * Response accuracy Startled (context * fear-potentiated)	Analgesia * Early developmental approach * Avoidance * Facial expression * Freezing * Open field * inhibitory control * Response time * Risk assessment * social approach	Fear survey schedule * SUDS	Behavioral approach test * CO_2 challenge test * Cold pressor test * Fear conditioning * Stranger tests * Trier social stress test

So far, the RDoC is only used in research settings, not in clinical practice. (It is hard to envision, as it is currently constituted, that it could be of practical clinical use.)

Source: Science-Based Medicine, (https://science basedmedicine.org/ dms/-5-and-the-fight-for-the-heart-of-psychiatry/. Steven Novella, M.D.)

Dr. Novella is a neurologist at the Yale University School of Medicine. He diagnoses and treats a wide variety of neurological conditions. He also is responsible for a blog, NeuroLogicaBlog, which covers a wide variety of topics, neuroscience, general science, philosophy of science, and the intersection of science with the media and society.

Dr. Novella brings his perspective to the criticism of the DSM-5. He duly notes NIMH Director Thomas Insel: "The goal of this new manual (the DSM) is to provide a common language for describing psychopathology. Dr. Insel acknowledges that the DSM does have reliability in that clinicians use the same terms to discuss clinical matters, but unlike in medicine, it lacks validity. Diagnoses like ischemic heart disease, lymphoma, or AIDS are based on objective criteria, laboratory results, or findings on imaging studies. Psychiatric diagnoses, on the other hand, are based on consensus about clusters of clinical symptoms, not any objective laboratory measure..."

Of course, Dr. Novella notes this, but he also brings to the DSM discussion a broader perspective. It is not as if psychiatry is less scientific than other medical specialties; it is only traveling a road that all medical specialties have followed in the past as they developed. He comments that it is part of the understanding of any disease that at first, it is the symptoms and signs that are apparent. The next phase, understanding the pathophysiology, comes gradually as research continues. Amyotrophic lateral sclerosis (ALS) was first seen as progressive muscle weakness. Later, it was learned that the weakness is caused by the destruction of a particular class of cells, motor neurons. The cause, however, is still unclear. Another neurological disorder, migraine headaches, is still largely diagnosed on the basis of symptoms—the location, description, frequency, and intensity. Multiple sclerosis is described by what is known about its pathophysiology. Criticizing the DSM-5 because it is still diagnosing mental disorders by presenting symptoms is medically necessary until there is gathering pathophysiological information to permit a transition, as has occurred in many other medicine specialties. He feels the NIMH, by declaring the DSM to be "flawed," is taking an extreme position. He uses the term "placeholder," which applies to the DSM until research delineates biological markers, hopefully as soon as possible. Indeed, "an evidence-based overhaul is needed, but it probably will meet resistance from the 'old guard.'" (He must be referring to the psychiatric profession.)

He observes there are certain differences between psychiatric disorders and medical disorders. "The NIMH claim that all mental disorders are biological is overly simplistic. Mental disorders are a complex combination of brain function and environmental factors. We will therefore never get completely away from clinical criteria, even if they are better informed by biological information" (This author also wants to include the cognitive, emotional, and even some psychodynamic components of these illnesses.)

Dr. Novella is enthusiastic about a prospective new approach moving away from the DSM and in the direction advocated by the NIMH. The emphasis on genetics, imaging, and laboratory research is made possible by advances in technology.

The effort is to identify networks and modules in the brain that are associated with symptoms. In genetics, a cluster of gene variants have been shown to increase the risk of developing autism spectrum disorders.

Psychiatry has lagged behind other medical specialties because "the subject matter is genuinely complex," but eventually, generic and neuroscientific information will "transform the field and our thinking about mental disorders." He ends, "The DSM is a necessary placeholder, but that means its reign must end one day."

Is Psychiatry a Medical Specialty?

Certainly, the expectation in the United States is that there will be reasonable access to a medical provider in all medical specialties, i.e., to a family physician, internist, general surgeon, etc. But what of psychiatrists, supposedly the frontline physicians for so-called "mental" health disorders? Theresa Ngvyen, LCSW, describes her experiences in making referrals to psychiatrists:

Source: "The Lack of Psychiatrists, Just One Barrier to Treatment." https://www.psycom.net/inside_americas-psychiatrist_shortage . (A devastating void)

Nguyen describes her experience referring children to psychiatrists in the Washington D.C. area in a relatively well-off community. Children discharged from a hospital mental health program could not be scheduled sooner than four months or longer. "The need was urgent, but no one was available. The shortage is so significant it's affecting everyone, regardless of income level." She gives some individual examples. A postpartum mom with severe depression took her life because the nearest appointment was three months away. A college student, away from home, was completely unable to make an appointment at his school's behavioral health center because it no longer was taking patients. A forty-two-year-old depressed man turned his gun on himself because the soonest appointment, for which he would have to drive four hours, was in three weeks. She quotes a report from the Kaiser Family Foundation, published in *The Journal of the American Medical Association* in 2017, which noted the "disease burden" from mental health or substance abuse is as great as that for cancer or heart disease, "but just 40 percent of adults and 50 percent of children" receive any mental health treatment. The most common reason is the "yawning 'psychiatrist gap.'"

Another paper, a 2018 report, "The Silent Shortage: A White Paper Examining Supply, Demand, and Recruitment Trends in Psychiatry," by Merritt Hawkins, a large physician-search firm, determined that there are nine psychiatrists per 100,000 people, an inadequate number, which should be at least fifteen, to provide mental health care services. The availability of psychiatric services varies enormously by region. Some parts of New York State have an estimated 612 psychiatrists per 100,000 population, but there is less than one per 100,000 in Idaho. In Texas, of the total number of counties, 254 lack a psychiatrist. The availability of psychiatric services will be diminished further due to refinements. Sixty percent are over fifty-five. Research has been conducted, called "mystery shoppers," to determine waiting times for an evaluation. Benzion Blech, MD, in "A Devastating Void of Service Availability," described the findings of the neurology department at the Mayo Clinic and associate researchers. They called one hundred fifty psychiatrists to schedule an evaluation in 2017 in the Washington D.C. area. Just 15 percent were accepting new patients, and only 7 percent had availability within two weeks. In another mystery shopper study, conducted for a Maryland health plan, out of 1,154 psychiatrists, only 14 percent were accepting new patients in the next forty-five days. In the Los Angeles area, 229 psychiatrists in the County Super Pages were contacted and told the prospective symptoms patients had "serious" mental health symptoms who needed a medication evaluation. Just twenty-eight appointments could even be scheduled, and 80 percent of them had to wait five weeks. The author also notes that "for those with severe problems, in-patient programs are shrinking." So-called mental health insurance companies limit coverage in a confusing way. Needed admission can be delayed for many days; evaluations are often superficial, with short visits and the absence of a detailed history, thoughtful diagnosis, and specific treatment plans. Also, the monitoring of medications is characterized by excessive intervals.

In much of the country, family doctors, physician assistants, and nurse practitioners attempt to supply needed mental health services as best they can. There is no other medical specialty in the United States, however, which offers less care for diagnosis and treatment.

There is a tremendous heterogenicity in the session lengths psychiatrists use for appointments with patients. The all-time championship for jamming in as many patients per hour as possible was a psychiatrist who saw forty. He was proud of his best day when he notched forty-seven. The only thing more outstanding than his speed was his psychopathy. One would hope he was to malpractice attorneys as honey is to bumblebees. Errors of omission in his practice would likely be as thick as the crust of barnacles on an old sailing vessel.

Then there are the ten-minute "med checkers" who see six patients per hour. Actual face time is perhaps five to seven minutes. An accurate label for such practitioners is that they run "medication mills."

The patient learns to start her interview as she is walking into the office. The practitioner has no time to listen. If the patient verbalizes that she is depressed, she is not asked why; instead, one antidepressant is prescribed. If a side effect is mentioned, there is no time to discuss it or provide a plan; only a quick medication maneuver occurs. Patients comment that such doctors only "tell" and don't listen. Psychiatry is supposed to abide by what is called the bio-psycho-social model—that is, to understand that symptoms occur in the context of environments and relationships. No time to open up that can of beans! Nor to explore lifestyle issues or stressors or educate about pharmacology. One can definitely claim that in such sessions, thorough, meaningful assessments are impossible; the patient is reduced to a symptom and chemicals. And often, the process of making a diagnosis is superficial and slapdash, just choosing one for purpose of insurance reimbursement. And then there are the psychiatrist "sages," seeing each patient for a so-called full session of forty-five minutes weekly. This is by far the preferred style of practice for the great majority of psychiatrists. The objective is to "remodel" patients' characters. And indeed, that may be beneficial for some patients, but who and how is often a mystery. These psychiatrists are usually poorly informed about neuroscience and sophisticated psychopharmacology. Given the severe shortage of psychiatric services, however, this type of practice seriously limits the number if patients who receive effective diagnosis and treatment.

Perhaps the best compromise is the half-hour, twenty-five-to-thirty-minute appointment, which would follow an in-depth evaluation of at least sixty minutes.

A Review of the Book *Healing: Our Path from Mental Illness to Mental Health*, by Thomas Insel, MD

This is a comprehensive critique of the functioning of the mental health services available currently (2022) for people symptomatic due to "mental" illness. From the jacket cover, Dr. Insel is both a psychiatrist and neuoscientist. From 2002 to 2015, he was director of the

National Institute of Mental Health in Washington, D.C. Since May 2019, he has been a special advisor to Gavin Newsom, the governor of California. He is a member of the National Academy of Medicine and has been the recipient of many awards and honorary degrees in the US and Europe.

When he was still director at NIMH, he was giving a lecture when the father of a boy with schizophrenia yelled from the back of the lecture hall, "Our house is on fire, and you're telling me about the chemistry of the paint. When are you going to put out the fire?"

It just sunk in for him. The man was correct and also sounded desperate. That stirred him to leave NIMH and to survey "mental" health services in the United States himself. "The gargantuan American mental health industry was not healing millions who were desperately in need of help." His book is a summary of his findings about mental health care.

And what he found was a "crisis of care, over and over again. I heard providers on the front lines describe mental health care in this country as a crisis." Families with an ill child or relative "told me about their desperate efforts to find a place to go in an emergency or their frustrating search to find effective care for a loved one with a complex illness that an antidepressant didn't help," and even more discomforting, "current treatments work; mental illness is not a life sentence; people can recover. I saw again and again programs, practitioners, and individuals achieving this goal of healing and recovery."

Within the "mental" health arena, among the various types of therapists, MSWs and PhDs, it is only the MD psychiatrist who can do the prescribing of "psychotropic" medication, although psychiatry itself prescribes for only 20 percent, the minority of patients who receive any prescription medication for "mental" symptoms. They have managed to "offload" 80 percent of their "mental" patients onto primary care practitioners, who do *not* have specialized training in the class of psychotropic medications. This while they go about employing character-building, extremely deep, time-consuming emotional-conflict

alleviating, and uncovering psychodynamic psychotherapy, obviously far more important for the well-being of their patients than mere
"medication." (Those meds—let the GPs do them. That 80 percent,
out of sight, out of mind.) This is unique to psychiatry.

Psychiatry's approach can be contrasted with the practice of neurologists who offload their equivalent of psychotherapy, physical therapy, to trained non-MD physical therapists while, like all other medical specialties, concentrating on the medical side of their specialty,
especially pharmacology (medication).

But perhaps it makes no difference to the psychiatrist's "mental
cases," because psychotropic medications are less effective than other types, such as cardiac or neurological medications. To quote Dr.
Insel, "There is an intense and continuing debate about the value of
psychiatric medications, a debate which is infrequent in other areas
of medicine." (That sentence alone will lower the confidence of those
who receive a prescription. And it's certainly true, when the officials
who evaluate all medications at the FDA, when they are evaluating a
psychotropic type, automatically lower their standards to allow at least
some of them to be marketed.)

And as to the nature of so-called "mental" illnesses, Dr. Insel explains, "I use the term 'mental illness' to refer to disorders of the mind,
manifested as changes in how we think, feel and behave." He continues, there is "not (yet) an identifiable lesion." His conclusion that
"mental" illness is all in the "mind" certainly is compatible with the
psychiatric practice of psychoanalytic psychotherapy, but isn't apoptosis and it's dysregulation (hyperapoptosis) and brain atrophy occurring
in the actual brain of the severely mentally ill a physically identifiable
lesion? It is a mystery that the good doctor makes no mention of those
damaging physical processes! (They *are* actually occurring in the brain!
They are damaging the brain, and only indirectly, due to decrements
of function, the "mind.")

No other medical specialty so fastidiously ignores the dysfunctions of the physical organ they (don't) study. But for psychiatry, their

pervasive preoccupations are the "mind" and the "psyche." Freud, who lacked the technology to find the true causation of "mental" illness in his era, would be attracted like a moth to a light to our modern technology, which has elucidated the physical brain dysregulations etiological to the misnamed "mental" illnesses.

Overall, Dr. Insel's book (which, in the opinion of this author, does mislead in the matter of "just medication," and "There is no lesion," surveys in detail the lapses, blind spots, and gross inefficiencies in the "mental" healthcare system. If it were hung in a closet as a suit, it would be moth-eaten and unfit to wear.)

Clinical Psychopharmacology

Somehow, Dr. Insel never even mentions this new medical specialty. The reader of his book would only glean an unfavorable opinion about "just medication." It has its own journal, specialty organization, and several textbooks. It's unclear where the good doctor has been? But you'll learn nothing about it from his book. It is a specialty still in development, but ultimately should be the successor to psychiatry, which, along with neurology, will be the two medical specialties focused on that important organ, the *brain*! The two specialties both overlap but also have separate domains of interest. Both use the procedures and processes of clinical medicine.

ALL-184

Dr. Insell expresses a great admiration for the pharmacological protocols developed for the treatment of "ALL" (acute lymphoblastic leukemia), a dreaded illness afflicting youngsters two to five years of age. In the 1970s, it was 90 percent fatal. The treatments were almost as horrible as the disease. Over the next forty years, sophisticated medicinal protocols employing combinations of the same medications available in the 1970s have resulted in a dramatic turnaround, with a 90 percent survival rate. Dr. Insel summarizes, "Continual improvement of the drug protocols, the nursing protocols, the surveillance— this is what success required. Not a breakthrough, but a relentless pursuit that combined available treatment for long-term recovery, not short-term remission." The success of ALL, he comments, "is important to remember for mental illness." And the changes and innovations he outlines for mental health treatment are contained in his comprehensive book.

Interestingly, what Dr. Insel misses is that "just medication," in the form of clinical psychopharmacology, actually has the potential to simulate ALL to some degree, because like ALL, it employs complex combinations of medications that have the potential to systematize the pharmacological treatment of so-called mental disorders. A new specialty "pregnant" with potential.

This author took a full four-day course presented by Massachusetts General Hospital and the Harvard Department of Psychiatry, the "44th Annual Psychopharmacology Conference—Live Stream Conference." Material was presented from 8:30 a.m. to 8:30 p.m.(During such a large segment of time, they were certainly discussing more than "just medication.")

The following list of contents at the conference is not presented for the reader to memorize, but just to convey an impression of the breadth of topics.

Program Agenda

Law and Psychiatry
Psychometric Medicine-Consults
The Neuroscience Revolution
Bipolar Depression
Bipolar Long-Term Management
Treatment Resistant Depression
PTSD
Anxiety Disorders and Treatments
Mood and Anxiety Disorders in
Pregnancy. Course and Treatment
Postpartum Mood Disorders
Natural Medications for Psychi-
atric Disorders
Suicide
The Neurobiology of Mood and
Psychotic Disorders
Psychopharmacology of Sleep
Disorders
The Neurobiology of Mood and
Psychotic Disorders
Cognitive Behavioral Therapy to
Augment Pharmacology
Psychedelic Medicine
First Episode Psychosis and
Schizophrenia
Management, Side-Effects of
Antipsychotics
Ketamine and Esketamine From
Recent Clinical Practice

Cognitive-Behavioral Therapy to
Augment Psychopharmacological
Treatment
Psychedelic Medicine
First Episode Psychosis and
Schizophrenia
Management, Side-Effects, Anti-
psychotics
Ketamine and Esketamine, From
Recent Clinical Practice
Stimulation and/or Surgical Ap-
proaches to Psychiatric Illness
New Treatments in Schizophrenia
New Treatments in Mood Dis-
orders
What is New in Addition?
Geriatrics
Traumatic Brain Injury
Illuminating the Black Box, An-
tidepressants, Youth and Suicide
PMDD and Depression, Meno-
pause, Transition, New Insights
Alcohol and Opiates
Tobacco and Cocaine
OCD
CBT for OCD
Pediatric Bipolar Disorders
ADHD
Drug Interactions

Stigma

The Biggest Cause of Stigma Is the Classification of Major Depression, Bipolar Disorder, and Schizophrenia as *"Mental!"*

Would you ordinally slur another? Psychiatrists, you would think, would be most sensitive to the nuances, the unconscious impact of certain expressions, and the intrapsychic stress they provide. Most psychiatrists would never resort to using ethnic, religious, or racial slurs. Yet when it comes to their own bailiwick, they are surprisingly dense, throwing about the word "mental," oblivious to its associated unconscious connotations. "Mental" illness, "mental" cases, "mental" health, "mental" health treatment, "mental," "mental," "mental!" Does the use of the frame of reference produce attraction, confidence, an urge to assume that label for oneself? Does it facilitate motivation to accept an illness and seek "mental health" treatment?

Let's just face facts! Organized psychiatry is a self-interested group that, above all, is interested in protecting their remuneration, which is derived mostly from weekly psychotherapy with each of their patients. They have to keep the terminology "mental." Psychotherapy is a "talking" modality that is "mental" in its essence. As long as psychiatrists are habituated to earning money in that way, they will *never* be willing to change the classification of these illnesses, which in their true nature are *physical* brain illnesses. They are not "mental"…slur… slur…illnesses.

The True Meaning of the Term "Mental Illness"

In his book *Healing: Our Path from Mental Illness to Mental Health*, Dr. Insel discusses the impact of stigma on attitudes toward these illnesses and psychiatric treatments. (Although he never deviates from the Holy Grail of the "mental" classification.)

The actress Glenn Close was sitting on a stool on an empty stage. But what she said, Insel thought, "I will never forget." In a flat tone of voice, she intoned, "I have a mental illness." He could only assume most of the audience would automatically and instantaneously, probably at an unconscious level, react with fear, being repelled. After a brief silence, she then added, "in my family." He suspected the audience, relieved, would then respond with empathy and compassion.

He quotes a young man who survived a dive off the San Francisco-Oakland Bay Bridge, alias the Golden Gate: "I had to decide. Do I want to kill myself, or do I want to see a psychiatrist? I hated myself enough to want to die, but not so much that I would become a mental patient!" (Suicide survivor, quoted by Suicide Prevention Task Force, 2014).

He refers to an article written many years ago in the *New Yorker* magazine. The author, Tad Friend, wrote an article entitled "Jumpers." He interviewed twenty-six people who made the jump off the Golden Gate but survived. In almost all cases, the four-second descent was accompanied by a radical change of perspective, leading to second thoughts! (And they're the very lucky ones!)

In his long sojourn interviewing patients and families, Insel determined that "in nearly every conversation, they pointed to 'stigma' as the biggest problem in mental health." This is a prejudice with several tentacles. It is why there is inadequate insurance coverage, inadequate funding for research, and the failure to improve treatment outcomes. "The diagnosis of a mental illness is freighted with emotion." He refers to the "complicated experience of having a mental illness." A symptom of some of the very ill is a loss of judgment and insight and the denial of illness (their brains are no longer under voluntary control). Plus, they also absorb the biases and prejudices of the general society, a "cultural hostility" toward the so-called "mentally" ill. So, in addition to the symptomatic misery and failures of function, they are encumbered, unlike those who are classified as "physically" ill, with the burden of a dark cloud of bias and rejection.

And therefore, we shouldn't be surprised if psychiatric treatment suffers from the same low opinion. Even Dr. Insell himself seems to have been afflicted with a prejudice against psychiatric medication when it came to his eight-year-old son (and he a senior psychiatrist and neuroscientific researcher). When his son was diagnosed with ADHD, he thought of psycho-social treatments, a special school, psychotherapy, and parent training. About having him treated with stimulant medication (considered the pharmacological treatment of choice), "Our whole-grain no sugar eight-year-old on a psychotropic drug, no way!" Finally, his resistance was lowered to pharmacological treatment after consulting with a child psychiatrist friend who recommended a "pilot" trial of methylphenidate (Ritalin). "Within a few hours, we watched our whirling dervish son slowdown, put his toys away and begin to listen for the first time…We were stunned."

This author has two observations: Most parents do not have a friendly, knowledgeable colleague to chat with informally before the decision to start a medication. It's surely handy to have a friendly, trusted colleague on the spot to mitigate your own prejudices, and Dr. Insel, based on the obvious improvement of his son, because of his "trial" on methylphenidate, jumps to a very general conclusion: "This response remains one of the most convincing statements I have ever heard about psychopharmacology!" Actually, if his son's response was written up in scientific literature, it would be a "case report." A case report, by itself (the doctor should know this), can never result in a definitive conclusion of efficiency for a class of medication in general medicine or psychiatry, let alone an entire field of practice (psychopharmacology).

And if Dr. Insel, after forty professional years in psychiatry, was so trepidatious to treat his son with a stimulant, what torments many parents must undergo in the matter of treating their own children with ADHD. (Please refer to chapter which reviews the FDA's procedures for evaluating efficacy and safety of all medications in the United States before they can be marketed.) This author does wonder if Dr. Insel is familiar with FDA data. If he were, he could have readily researched the scientific data on the efficacy and side-effect profile for methylphenidate. Unfortunately, from the tone of his discussion on stimulant therapy, the anxieties and uncertainties of parents facing a similar decision as he did with his eight-year-old son, after reading his comments about methylphenidate, will only have their anxieties exacerbated, not assuaged. If Dr. Insel were only a junior resident in training, his comments would not result in untoward circumstances, but he is the epitome of stature and seniority in psychiatry. And his book, broadcasting his status and expertise, which has a colorful cover jacket and multiple endorsements, will probably have a wide audience. Its target audience is the general public (including all those parents with ADHD-compromised offspring). Come to think about it, he could have changed the tone of his book if, instead of sharing his own bias, he had reviewed for his readers the *actual* scientific data for stimulant treatment for ADHD. (Although unlike him, they may suffer additional trials and tribulations in trying to locate a competent diagnostician and prescriber.)

And of course, in recommending treatment with psychotropics, the same barrier of stigma and bias weighs on it. Since psychiatry had "foisted" 80 percent of these treatment encounters onto the backs of primary care providers while the bulk of their time is devoted to time-consuming, deep, deep weekly psychotherapy to build new personalities, obviously, commitment to develop true expertise in clinical psychopharmacology is limited. Like the appendix, it is a vestigial enterprise to them. And the primary care doctors are occupied with multiple (less important) "physical" illnesses, which, of course, can never accomplish a rebuilding of a patient's entire personality. The family doctors do not have the training to administer complex psychopharmacology or even to diagnose patients who may need it. Now, it's not entirely hopeless. Perhaps 10-15 percent of psychiatrists do make the effort to develop competence in clinical psychopharmacology. Good luck in selecting a psychiatrist with documented expertise in it.[37] (But Russian roulette can be interesting, if not always beneficial).

As we have seen, even an experienced psychiatrist can have a latent bias toward psychiatric medications, so you can only imagine the bias in the public mind. He describes a feature story about patterns of medication use in the British newspaper *The Guardian*. Medication for common medical illnesses, antihypertensives, cholesterol medications, and others provoked no controversy, but when antidepressants were reviewed, there was a loud clamor that people were being "drugged." And of course, ECT is the poster child for stigmatization (perhaps approaching the stigma of "the rack" used for torture in the Middle Ages). ECT grossly underutilized in the United States in spite of over eighty scientific studies attesting to its efficacy and safety. The only institutions that do utilize it for severe major depression are the highest-quality medical centers: Harvard, Yale, Columbia, Johns Hopkins, etc. (Someone at those institutions must actually have read the scientific literature on ECT!)

Overall, Dr. Insel's book does pull out the moth-eaten suit that represents the current so-called "mental" healthcare system, for a thorough inspection. It is not known, however, if there are any willing and competent tailors in the vicinity.

"Anti-Psychiatry"

Who are these people who habitually "vent their spleen" at psychiatry? Some appear to be in the grip of a particular passion that agitates them so, and which is directed exclusively at psychiatry and no other branch of medicine. One wonders what is egging them on.

It is a movement that perceives psychiatric diagnosis and treatment as fundamentally unscientific, promoting more harms than

---

37   One possible guide might be to inquire what the psychiatrist has chosen for his continuing education requirements mandated by the AMA or APA. Are they centered on pharmacology and neuroscience?

benefits—indeed, that there are incidents of "extreme" harms from electroconvulsive therapy, involuntary commitment, and drugs, particularly antipsychotics. Actually, 80 percent of antidepressant drugs are prescribed by primary care physicians, and much of the rest of their armamentarium involving anticonvulsants prescribed for bipolar spectrum mood disorders are also prescribed by neurologists for various types of seizure disorders. Well, the anti-psychiatry skeptics could postulate seizures are obviously "physical" in contrast to mood illnesses, but some forms of epilepsy, absence seizures, lack an obvious disturbance of movement.

The Rosenhan Experiment

A very enterprising psychologist, David Rosenhan, a professor at Stanford University, designed an elaborate experiment[38] to study the validity of psychiatric diagnosis in 1973. The result appeared in the journal *Science*, titled "On Being Sane in Insane Places."

He and seven "mentally healthy" individuals presented themselves to a total of twelve psychiatric hospitals on the West Coast, claiming they were hearing voices (having auditory hallucinations). They were all admitted. Once admitted, they were instructed to deny any further hallucinations and report feeling normal. Expect for one being diagnosed as having bipolar disorder, the rest were diagnosed as schizophrenic. None of the staff identified them as being imposters, but interestingly, thirty-five of a total of 118 of the hospitalized patients identified them as not being genuine patients, instead thinking they were researchers or journalists investigating the hospital. It was left for the "pseudo-patients" to get out of the hospital using their own devices. Before discharge, they all had to agree to continue the prescribed antipsychotic medication after discharge, and presumably, follow-up was arranged with outpatient prescribers. None of the pseudo-patients had actually taken the antipsychotic medication in the

---

38   Antipsychiatry, Wikipedia. The Rosenhan experiment.

hospital, instead flushing their doses. The average duration of stay was nineteen days.

There was an additional study, "The Nonexistent Imposter Experiment," also in 1973. During a three-month period, 193 patients (none were "pseudo-patients") were admitted to a selected psychiatric service. Beforehand, the staff had been prepped that some of them would be imposters. The staff judged that forty-one were suspect. To their credit, psychiatrists made that judgement only nineteen times, for an error rate of around 10 percent (which is probably not dissimilar to general medical diagnosis).

Rosenhan, in his article in *Science* about the studies, took issue that psychiatric diagnosis is specific or reliable. "Any diagnostic pacer that lends itself to readily to massive errors of this sort cannot be a very reliable one."

Rosenhan's conclusions did draw forth a critique. A prominent professor of psychiatry, Dr. Robert Spitzer, on the staff of Columbia Presbyterian Medical Center, noted a response to Rosenhan's article by another accomplished psychiatrist, Seymour S. Kety, M.D.:

"If I were to drink a quart of blood and, concealing what I had done, come to the emergency room of any hospital vomiting blood, the behavior of the staff would be quite predictable. If they labeled and treated me as having a bleeding peptic ulcer, I doubt that I could argue convincingly that medical science does not know how to diagnose that condition."

He pointed out that physicians do not assume patients are dissembling or malingering about symptoms upon initial contact, and it should not be assumed psychiatrists conclude that a patient does not have a mental illness either. He concluded that Rosenhan's study, "lacked realism."

In 2019, author Susannah Cahalan, in her book *The Great Pretender*, wrote about her review of Rosenhan's documents, which he had left behind after his death. She found that his article in *Science* was based on "inconsistent data, misleading descriptions, and inaccurate or fabricated quotations from psychiatric records."

In 2008, the BBC's science program *Horizon* concluded a similar experiment entitled "How Mad Are You?" Ten subjects were utilized, five having a "mental health" diagnosis, the other five with no such history. Three experts in mental health diagnosis were requested to distinguish among them based on just their behavior, but no other input. The "experts" correctly diagnosed only two and misdiagnosed another two as mentally ill, who weren't.

This author has two responses. Whatever the diagnostic criticism, there is no doubt that some individuals suffer horribly and have destroyed lives due to these afflictions, and that the BBC's so-called "experiment" is vacuously nonsensical. No physician, including psychiatrists, makes a diagnosis just by looking at a patient.

The greatest consternation that agitates the anti-psychiatrists is forced or involuntary treatment. (They are clueless that severe mental illnesses, i.e., a person with a schizophrenic episode or another with bipolar disorder in a manic crisis, is subjected to such powerful, agonizing symptoms on an involuntary basis, and these illnesses wreak havoc on the normal functioning of their wills.) They ignore these clear clinical facts. For such afflicted people, the anti-psychiatrists will be happiest if those people are *free* to die with their boots on in the midst of an agonizing symptomatic storm.

Thomas Szasz, the author of the 1961 book, *The Myth of Mental Illness*, was the most prominent spokesman of the anti-psychiatry perspective even though he was a psychiatrist who also had psychoanalytic training. He postulated that insanity was not a medical but a moral issue. (All the more reason for the seriously "medically" ill to feel degraded.) A trio of "mental" health professionals, Franco Basaglia, Giorgio Antonucci, and Bruce E. Levine asserted that psychiatry used psychiatric hospitals to "control and medicalize deviant behaviors and social problems...on behalf of the existing establishment." Certain organizations, MindFreedom International and the World Network

Users, assert that psychiatrists exaggerate the claim that their medications are effective and minimize very serious side effects. For example, stimulants prescribed for children induce abnormal movements, spasms, and tics and also impose "unjust social control." Peter Breggin, actually a psychiatrist and the author of several books, including *Toxic Psychiatry*, highlights the pernicious role of the pharmaceutical companies by means of what are essentially bribes, sponsoring dinners at expensive restaurants, distributing gifts, and even paying for weekend trips to fancy resorts, although regulations have now somewhat limited the pharmaceutical industry's endeavors to enhance the volume of prescriptions for their particular drugs.

And the utilization of ECT gives the anti-psychiatrists conniption fits. The major teaching hospitals: Harvard, Yale, Columbia Presbyterian, etc., however, have ECT services. Perhaps they are torturers in disguise.

The act of committing patients to a psychiatric hospital or a psychiatric unit in a general hospital is felt by the anti-psychiatrists to be quite grisly, as if the committed patient were being thrust into a snake pit from which there will be no escape. It is seen by them "as a violation of the fundamental principles of free or open societies." And as in any ideological movement, there are the fanatical extremists, those who unambiguously argue for the complete elimination of psychiatry.

A few notes on the actual nature of involuntary commitment are in order. The committed patient does not spend an eternity in a snake pit. In a well-ordered psychiatric unit, the objective is to ameliorate symptoms as soon as possible with a minimum of force. Involuntary commitment is always accompanied by a visit from an attorney to assess the patient's status. Generally, the patient improves and signs in on a voluntary basis. If the patient is still severely symptomatic, after a short period, the attorney will present him/her in court. The judge will make the decision about discharge or further mandated hospitalization until a further court appearance if required.

The anti-psychiatry movement lives on. On October 7, 2016, the Ontario Institute for Studies in Education at the University of Toronto announced the establishment of a scholarship for students writing theses on the anti-psychiatry movement.

Every organization protects its turf, including professional organizations. In this article "The Battle for the Soul of Psychiatry."[39] Dr. Awais Aftab, MD, interviews Ronald W. Pies, MD, Professor Emeritus of Psychiatry at SUNY-Upstate Medical Center and Clinical Professor of Psychiatry at Tuft University School of Medicine. He is the author or coauthor of several psychiatric textbooks. The subject is the criticisms directed toward psychiatry, of which Dr. Pies is an articulate defender.

The gold standard of practice for psychiatrists is traditional "psychoanalytically" oriented psychotherapy. It involves seeing each patient for a forty-five-minute appointment at least on a weekly basis, often more. It is a comfortable mode of practice for them, permitting them to keep their patient rosters very low relative to other medical specialties while maintaining a reliable, consistent income stream. They promote their psychotherapy as "medical" to distinguish it from the psychotherapy of psychologists and social workers, thus warranting significantly higher charges.

But it is the least-scrutinized form of psychotherapy. Cognitive behavioral therapy, utilized by psychologists, has been scientifically studied and is therefore "evidence-based," but no one can really say what's going on in the psychiatrists' offices. Whatever it is, it is totally dependent on the individual technique of each psychiatrist. It is a totally private affair, and even after a year or two of therapy, patients may be confused about therapeutic goals and progress, as there is little structure or specific goal-setting. There is no doubt that some psychiatrists do provide a genuine service, but overall, the entire business is highly subjective.

Perhaps over time, the weekly discussion is helpful, or it could just be a form of expensive conversation continued for two, three, or more years. Who knows?

---

39 The Battle for the Soul of Psychiatry https://www.psychiatrictimes.com June 24, 2020. Awais Aftab M.D.

But "turf-protection" is the real issue, and that involves defending against the assault by the "anti-psychiatry" movement (of all the medical specialties, only psychiatry has this responsibility, as to date, there are no anti-neurology, anti-dermatology, or anti-internal medicine movements).

Dr. Aftab initiates the interview by observing, "Psychiatry has been under attack for so long now that many psychiatrists are quite weary of the critique." Dr. Pies describes some of the most extreme critics; they are hostile "and use vituperative rhetoric which is clearly aimed at discrediting psychiatry as a medical discipline." The article quotes Dr. Nassir Ghaemi, a prominent academic psychiatrist, about the anti-psychiatry movement, which is "that movement which denies the fundamental legitimacy of psychiatry as a medical specialty, consistently imputes malign or mendacious motives to the profession, and which denies the efficacy and legitimacy of psychiatric treatment, particularly somatic treatments."

Dr. Pies amplifies that they make "bogus arguments and hateful attacks" in which they "fallaciously marginalize psychiatry from the other medical specialties."

Another issue of great concern is how so-called "mental" illness is being attributed to a "chemical imbalance" in the brain. (This is particularly threatening to psychiatrists because if the lesion is primarily "physical," there would be little rationale for psychiatrists continuing psychoanalytically oriented psychotherapy, for which a "psychological" etiology serves as a justification of medical necessity).

Dr. Pies expresses foreboding that the "chemical imbalance trope has become deeply ingrained among many in the general public," promulgated by the pharmaceutical industry and market forces. He clarifies that psychiatry has never considered it a "bona fide therapy." But that isn't stopping those current trends, which psychiatrists must resist, or they will be confined to doing brief "med checks." Psychotherapeutic services being handed off to non-physicians.

He explains that in his own department of psychiatry at SUNY Upstate Medical University, the integration of psychopharmacology and psychotherapy is taught and that the causes of mental illness are complex, with not just biological but also psychological and social roots—in other words, a bio-psycho-social theory.

Dr. Pies reviews a number of other concerns that "people with mental illness have indeed been marginalized and stigmatized, and so have those of us who care for them."

He observes that in contradiction to anti-psychiatry's nullification of the effectiveness of psychiatric treatment, and particularly the antagonism to the prescription of antipsychotics, antipsychotics definitely have "short-to-intermediate-term efficacy, six months to two years... in preventing relapse in schizophrenia." The evidence for that "is very compelling based on numerous studies." About antipsychotics, considerable controlled evidence shows that antipsychotic treatment improves quality of life by various measures." He educates that what anti-psychiatry criticizes—that antipsychotics lead to severe withdrawal symptoms— are actually the symptoms of the recurrence of the underlying disease, with no direct link to withdrawal phenomena."

Nevertheless, the critics "completely dismiss the therapeutic value of these medications" He summarizes about anti-psychotic medication, "Those of us who have spent our professional lives treating "the sickest of the sick"—patients whose lives have been destroyed by schizophrenia—"have little doubt that antipsychotic medication, judiciously prescribed, can literally be lifesaving. Armchair critics of the research literature are no substitute for working closely year after year with suffering patients and their families."

Dr. Pie also discusses two additional concerns:

One is that a distinction should be made between a transitory depression of mood in reaction to a stressful occurrence and a major depressive episode, which may be also triggered by a stressful occurrence. The latter should not be confused as a "problem in living," as it is a bona fide disease state usually associated with severe distress and often with degrees of incapacitation for which there is scientifically ev-idence–based treatment (if, by happenstance, it might be accessible).

Also, he draws a clear distinction between diagnosed "mental" ill-nesses and criminality. In particular, the media are always identifying serial murderers as "mentally" ill when they know little or nothing about their past histories. They just assume they're "mentally" ill. In the absence of competent diagnosis, such premature and amateurish pronouncements only perpetrate stigma.

"Serotonin or not, Antidepressants Work, Psychiatric Times, September 1022, Vol 39, No 09. Ronald W. Pies, MD: George Dawson, MD

They react to a recent article by British researchers Moncrieff, et al.[40] The article refutes the notion that major depressive disorder (MDD) is caused by lowered serotonin activity in the brain, the implication being that this is the primary cause of depression according to psychiatry. Follow-up articles extend their conclusions that given such a simplistic theory of etiology, the rationale for prescribing antidepressants is itself shaken. Their articles conclude the proclaimed benefit antidepressants have, and the specific mechanisms by which they alleviate depression is challenged: "Antidepressants appear to have a generalized emotion-numbing effect" (more or less like alcohol or phenobarbital), and "it is impossible to say that taking selective serotonin reuptake [SSRI] antidepressants is worthwhile...and it's not clear that SSRIs do more harm than good."

---

40   Moncrieff, J, Cooper RE, Stockman, T et al. The serotonin theory of depression: a systematic review of the evidence. Mol. Psychiatry. Published online, July 20, 2022.

And those conclusions are presented in this authoritative clinical (medical) journal read by prescribers, the majority being primary care practitioners as in the United States. In the conclusion of their article, Dr. Pies and Dawson express their wish: "We hope that patients and clinicians are not deterred from the use of antidepressants by the review (Moncrieff article)."

Under the Rubric, "Mental Illness-Mental Health"

Everyone is an "expert" in the field, in stark contrast to all other medical fields, from internal medicine to neurology, in which etiologies are, insofar as possible, based on scientifically designed studies and efficacy of treatment. Such studies are accepted as the definitive word. Similar studies in "mental" health and psychiatry, however, are paid little attention to. They are less interested in that than the joys derived from endlessly pontificating about the alleged shortcomings and defects of psychiatry.

In Table 1 of their article, they list seven reasons Moncrieff et al. have loaded injurious false information into their articles appearing in an authoritative journal.

1. Psychiatric authorities never held a theory that serotonin or other neurotransmitters are the exclusive causes of MDD.
2. "Psychiatrists have known for decades, the etiology…is extremely complicated…"
3. Moncrieff et al. ignored a large literature on the role of serotonin in MDD.

4. The report ignored four previous large studies that concluded there was little evidence serotonin was the primary etiological cause of MDD.

5. The brain contains up to seventy-five different neurotransmitters, so the conclusion that serotonin was the major etiological cause was never held by psychiatry.

6. For many *effective* drugs used in general medicine, neurology, and oncology, the mechanisms of action are unknown or not fully understood.

7. Similarly, for SSRIs, the precise mechanisms of action need not be fully understood in order to be effective in treatment.

What the widely distributed Moncrieff article probably did was to "turn off" the willingness of many prescribers to utilize SSRIs when they could relieve symptoms and reduce disabilities and suicide, making patients more reluctant to take them if they are prescribed by diminishing group of prescribers.

But "everyone" is an expert in "mental" health.

And now that Dr. Pies and Dawson have corrected the gross misinformation that depression is caused by a single neurotransmitter, a belief attributed to psychiatry by the Moncrieff articles, just what is the role of serotonin in the body?

"Serotonin: A Biography," Psychiatric Times.
September 2022. Vol. 39, No. 9. John J. Miller, MD

Judging from all the fuss about serotonin, you would think high gobs of it were confined to the brain and nowhere else in the body. Actually, 90 percent of serotonin is in the intestines and 8 percent in blood platelets, leaving only 2 percent for the entire brain. It is far more a "gut" chemical than a brain chemical. In the intestine, its main objective is to rid the body of any toxins that may have entered the intestinal tract. Colorfully named cells in the intestine, "enterochromaffin" cells, when they sense a toxin, secrete serotonin, designed to land on a specific serotonergic receptor, SHT-4, in the gut, which jacks up intestinal motility and secretions. Blood platelets, which store serotonin, also go on red-alert, secreting serotonin directly into the blood-fluid, which in turn reaches the brain, turning on serotonergic 5HT-3 receptors, which induce vomiting. So, our beloved molecule evacuates the poison from both ends of the gastrointestinal tracts. (So, if you swallow rat poison, make sure you have serotonin on board!)

In the brain, serotonin "has *some* involvement in complex processes," regulating mood and anxiety, sleep, cognition, temperature regulation, sexual drive, and appetite. In the past four decades, accumulating data has uncovered the existence of seven families of serotonergic receptors, which also have subfamilies. Pharmacological progress has resulted in medications that target and regulate particular receptors. Some examples: Ondansetron blocks the 5HT-3 receptor, relieving the symptoms of nausea. Triptan medications block the 5HT-1B and D receptors, relieving migraine headaches. Lorcaserin boosts the 5HT-2C receptor, promoting weight loss. But there is a nefarious role some other serotonergic receptors play, boosting the 5HT 2A receptor by hallucinogens psilocybin, LSD, and mescaline, can produce psychotic symptoms. Boosting the 5HT-2B receptors by fenfluramine or pergolide can cause the cardiac valves to lose flexibility and fibrose, resulting in serious heart disease.

Serotonin may have a more prominent role in treating anxiety symptoms and disorders than mood symptoms. The FDA approved SSRIs fluoxetine, sertraline, paroxetine, and fluvoxamine for treatment of obsessive compulsive disorder (OCD) in the late 1980s. SSRIs have demonstrated efficacy for the treatment of panic disorder, social anxiety disorder, and posttraumatic stress disorder.

A competent prescriber must be aware of potential side effects and monitor for them.

Milder side effects are fairly common. Severe adverse effects, thankfully, are rare, but the prescriber must be aware of them. Boosting the 5HT-3 and 5Ht-4 receptors can produce nausea, vomiting, abdominal cramping, and diarrhea. Platelet dysfunction can produce an increased bleeding tendency which could be problematic in certain medical disorders.

In summary, to quote from the article, "The human brain has 80 billion neurons. Each neuron has a synaptic connection to 10,000 other neurons. Hence, our brains have roughly 800 trillion synaptic connections...It would be naïve to believe that a single neurotransmitter, receptor or circuit in the brain will cure any psychiatric or neurological disorder...serotonin is just one letter in the encyclopedia of how the brain works."

Cognitive Behavioral Therapy

Even though the emphasis in this book has been on neuroscience and expert clinical psychopharmacology, certain evidence-based psychotherapies, if conducted by suitably trained and credentialed therapists, are part of the total armamentarium to relieve suffering and dysfunction produced by these illnesses. Cognitive behavioral therapy is the gold standard. This author took a yearlong postdoctoral fellowship in cognitive therapy procedures, but of the perhaps ten or twelve taking the training, there were no other psychiatrists; the rest were PhD's or postdoctoral MSWs. In other words, psychiatric-psychotherapy, by in large, is not evidence-based but rather a brew of various approaches and procedures, generally uncritiqued. In that brew, no doubt some psychiatrists are skilled therapists, but the naïve patient generally cannot know, in the beginning, which is which. So, psychotherapy rendered by psychiatrists is indeed a "mixed bag."

The Evaluation of the Therapist

In the case of a well-trained cognitive therapist, the psychotherapeutic tools and techniques have been carefully evaluated for efficacy and results in scientific studies and used in therapy as a standard protocol. There is a minimum of "mystery;" the patient can comprehend the techniques as he/she learns to use them. In other words, it is a "manualized" therapy, often in marked contrast to traditional psychiatric "psychoanalytic" psychotherapy, which rests solely on the authority and approach of a given psychiatrist, and indeed can veer off into the mysterious. And how is a patient to know of its effectiveness? Perhaps, after two years of weekly therapy, the patient may be able to make a determination? And the psychiatrist in a psychotherapeutic practice does not have the interest, willingness, or time to deal with the biological complexities of the brain and the related expert clinical psychopharmacology based on specific physical brain dysregulations. Seeing the average psychiatrist in his practice is a bit like playing Russian roulette. One of the six cartridges of the revolver might actually have a "golden" bullet—a psychiatrist skilled in psychotherapy based on his innate skills and training who also is an expert clinical psychopharmacologist.

Cognitive behavior training centers can be contacted to learn of qualified practitioners, who have trained there, but many practice in different states.

Beck Institute for Cognitive Behavior Therapy
Nonprofit organization
Beckinstitute.org

Beck Institute for Cognitive Behavior Therapy, a nonprofit organization located in suburban Philadelphia, is an international cognitive behavior therapy training and research center. It was founded in 1994 by Aaron T. Beck and his daughter Judith S. Beck. Aaron T. Beck was the Beck Institute's President Emeritus.

For information about specific topics, try one of these links:

- Questions about our training opportunities
- To schedule an appointment at the Beck Institute Clinic
- To subscribe to our Newsletter
- To obtain permission to use Beck Institute materials
- All other questions

One Belmont Avenue, Suite 503
Bala Cynwyd, PA 190041610
P: 610-664-3020
F: 610-709-5336
help@beckinstitute.org

Apoptosis/Hyperapoptosis

A question: Will Dr. Pies take hyperapoptosis (not yet termed a theory according to psychiatry) to the *woodshed* as he did for chemical imbalance theory (CIT)? The answer is not in. It is too soon. But hyperapoptosis as a biophysical pathological process occurring in at least three classes of so-called "mental" disorders: schizophrenia, bipolar disorder, and severe, recurrent major unipolar depression. Hyperapoptosis is not a *phantasmagoria*. Neurons in important brain areas like the hippocampi and the prefrontal cortex really do die at an abnormally accelerated rate, and the affected brain regions really do have a demonstrable loss of volume, i.e., "brain shrinking." The bio-psycho-social theory should continue to prevail, but the fact of a physical neurological pathology is occurring in these major "mental" disorders casts them in the mold of neurological-like disorders, like Alzheimer's disease, seizure disorders, Parkinson's disease, and multiple sclerosis. So far, psychiatry has not acknowledged the existence of this biophysical process as occurring in the forementioned disorders. Psychiatry tenaciously insists they are "mental" problems and that their patients are "mental cases," with the attendant stigmatization and humiliation of them. It is far-fetched to think they will reframe these illnesses as neurological-like, actually physical brain diseases, i.e., "neuriatric," removing the stigma of the "mental" classification, even though such a reclassification would promote enhanced prevention at all levels.

So unfortunately, the discordant methods of actual practice between psychiatry and neurology will continue even though they share the same certification organization, the American Board of Psychiatry and Neurology. Neurologists promptly use their medical expertise to intervene with pharmacology as the first line to combat hyperapoptosis. Psychiatrists leisurely search for "deep emotional conflicts," only a small minority emphasizing rapid diagnosis and expert pharmacological treatment. A thought experiment: What if neurologists practiced like the average psychiatrist, and instead of referring patients for physical therapy, they did it themselves? Their hard medical skills would atrophy, and their neurological pharmacotherapy skills would wither, preparing the groundwork for accelerated death of neurons (hyperapoptosis).

It has not been possible for this author to *poll* psychiatrists about their *familiarity* with hyperapoptosis. This author is not a librarian, but he was unable to locate any subject matter on it in the psychiatric literature or texts until finding one obscure article in a 2022 journal. (It should be noted that hyperapoptosis has been addressed in many nonpsychiatric journals since 1996. That's nearly *26 years*, but what psychiatrist reads those nonpsychiatric journals?) Neurologists diagnose and treat varieties of seizure disorders, some of which do not have apparent physical manifestations, such as absence seizures. If they practiced *like psychiatrists*, neurologists would have totally ignored that type of seizure for twenty-six years! (In spite of the fact that hyperapoptosis is most likely a relevant physical-pathological mechanism in epilepsy).

Just a brief review of hyperapoptosis. It is destructive to brain tissue (that's me being whittled away) resulting in significant, accelerated death of neurons (brain cells) before their time, thereby actually whittling away vital brain centers like the hippocampi (memory, learning, special sense) and the prefrontal cortex (judgment, insight, planning, managing). And the atrophy is visible on X-rays and scans. It's different than chemical imbalance theory (CIT). You can actually see the accumulated effects on scans. Also, there are emerging laboratory tests to measure hyperapoptosis. (A wager: that no psychiatrist has ever ordered such a test of living or dead patients!)

So as some of the patients of psychiatrists are losing their brains due to inadequate diagnosis and treatment, *what should be done?*

Last Chapter

Dr. Insel[41] has done something quite extraordinary. He set himself a project to thoroughly evaluate the results of "mental" health treatment in the United States and came up with a detailed appraisal of the efficiency of the system in terms of its impact on the status of patient well-being. His conclusion was blunt. The entire operation of the mental health care system does *not* improve outcomes for mental illnesses. That's really a shocker!

The question for this author is, what is psychiatry's contribution to this state of affairs? Does psychiatry play a role in or contribute to this miserable situation?

Something dramatic has occurred in the field of psychiatry, as yet not acknowledged by that specialty. Neuroscientific research and detailed imaging studies of the brain have demonstrated the major so-called "mental" illnesses, schizophrenia, bipolar disorders, and severe major depression are subject to dysregulated apoptosis in the same mode as neurological illnesses like Parkinson's disease, multiple sclerosis, and stroke. In common, the brain in all these illnesses feature hyperapoptosis. The result is accelerated death of neurons and brain shrinkage (atrophy). The consequence is worsening symptoms and incapacitation.

Neurology acknowledges this pathophysiological process and treats it with the best pharmacological treatments in its therapeutic

---

41 Healing. Our Path from Mental Illness to Mental Health. Thomas Insel, MD, Penguin Press.

armamentarium. Psychiatry, unfortunately, has not reached that stage. Neurology utilizes clinical neuropharmacology to the fullest. Eighty percent of psychiatrists are still in the "pill-prescribing" mode, i.e., writing an occasional prescription as an adjunct to psychotherapy, or in the five-to-ten-minute "med check" mode, not having sufficient time or knowledge to develop a comprehensive pharmacological strategy. Clinical psychopharmacology is not just a matter of dashing off a prescription. It is a new, full-blown medical specialty requiring specialized training and continual updating in continuing education, in a manner identical to internal medicine or neurology. There is a relatively new medical organization, the American Society of Clinical Psychopharmacology (ASCP), but only a small minority of psychiatrists have joined at this juncture. The ASCP is working on a means to certify in clinical psychopharmacology.

In view of the commonality of hyperapoptosis in schizophrenia, bipolar disorder, and severe major depression, the approach to these illnesses should be similar to clinical neuropharmacology for neurological disorders. Just pill-prescribing and psychoanalytic talking is inadequate, bordering on malpractice. The psychiatrist must be as proficient in clinical psychopharmacology as neurologists are in clinical neuropharmacology.

Yet only 15-20 percent of psychiatrists have met that standard, and the innocent layperson patient or prospective patient generally can't distinguish which psychiatrist is which.

What can psychiatrists do to improve outcomes?

(1) Open their minds that a physical, lethal biophysiological process, hyperapoptosis, is occurring in the major psychiatric illnesses, as it does in the major neurological illnesses.

(2) Respond appropriately to this process of accelerated death of precious neurons and brain shrinkage (atrophy).

(3) An appropriate response must be accelerated competent diagnosis and expert clinical psychopharmacological treatment.

(4) Emphasize in training programs and continuing education the primacy of expeditiously diagnosing the psychiatric illnesses in which hyperapoptosis is likely occurring and utilizing sophisticated psychopharmacology as the most likely, effective treatment.

(5) Realize that struggling to preserve the traditional psychotherapy format is a lost cause in terms of insurance-company coverage.

(6) But fight like mad to delegitimize the five-to-ten-minute "med check" as inherently a deficient form of treatment resulting in more harms than benefits to patients. (And first, do no harm.) This may require resorting to the courts.

(7) Instead, demand psychiatric sessions must be at minimum 25-30 minutes, for which insurance must reimburse at a reasonable fee level, or no more than two appointments per hour. This amount of time is critical to know the patient, learn what stressors are triggering symptoms and disabilities, develop clinical psychopharmacological strategies, and carefully monitor them. There are medical and societal costs to giving short shrift to patients with inadequate "med checks."

(8) As the neuroscientific revolution has documented, abnormal brain morphologies, numerous biochemical and neurotransmitter abnormalities, and genetic differences are the actual etiological basis for symptoms and incapacitations for schizophrenia, bipolar disorder, and major depression. It no longer is scientifically appropriate to designate them as "mental" illnesses. That classification has an overhang of serious stigma and humiliates patients unnecessarily. A new label should be considered to reclassify these illnesses, so they are not separated or isolated from all the other illnesses. Could an option be to relabel them "neuriatric" illnesses, with the root "neuro" shared with

neurology? This could only facilitate improvement in all levels of prevention. It would be such a relief to patients and prospective patients to lift from their shoulders the heavy burden of being labeled "mentally ill" or "mental cases." It is hard to imagine that twenty or fifty years from now, they would still be using such antiquated and stigmatizing terminology.

(9) Currently, 80 percent of patients with "mental" symptoms are never evaluated by a psychiatrist. This fact alone contributes to poor outcomes. Is there something wrong with a specialty that never interacts with 80 percent of its potential patients?

Patients, families and interested organizations have a direct interest in improving outcomes in the treatment of these disorders, which the author has suggested need a new classification to get away from the stigmatizing labels, "mental" illness, "mental" cases, that are inherently offensive and deter effective treatment. As we proceed into the twenty-first century, we should chuck the entire classification and turn to alternative labeling. This author has suggested the term, neuriatric, employing the same root, neuro, as in neurology. The disorders in the current DSM could be reclassified as cognitive, emotional, behavioral and personality dysregulations. So, no further "Diagnostic Statistical Manual of Mental Disorders." Instead,

"Diagnostic and Statistical Manual of Neuriatric Disorders and cognitive, emotional, behavioral and personality dysregulations."

Acknowledgments

Mrs. Etta Barmann of New York City Transcription patiently typed out the manuscript from my handwritten scrawls. I had heard Palmetto Publishing was an excellent company and was not disappointed. In particular, Grace Ardis and Kristin Graham were very responsive and helpful also their editing team for the review of the manuscript. Marci Friscia of Princeton Office Solutions facilitated necessary communications about the manuscript.

Bibliography

Marilyn Monroe Footnotes

Fn1 Marilyn Monroe. Wikipedia, pg17

Fn2 https://wwwbiography.com/news/marilyn-monroe-mother-rela-tionship. pg. 1.

Fn3 https://www.qcc.cuny.edu/socialscience/ppecorino/SS680/Fu-neral_Marilyn_Monroe.html

Fn4 The White Dress of Marilyn Monroe.WikipediaPg1 (2) ibid pg1. (3) ibid pg2. (4) ibid pg2.

Fn1 Marilyn

Legacy

Her Formative Years

The White Dress

Fn4 The White Dress of Marilyn Monroe.WikipediaPg1 (2) ibid pg1. (3) ibid pg2. (4) ibid pg2.

Forever Marilyn

Fn1 https://en.Wikpedia.org/wiki/ForeverMarilyn

Forever Marilyn in Australia and China

Fn1 Bendigo, Wikipedia

Fn1 "Marilyn Monroe exhibition a big splash for Bendigo tourism."abc.net.all

Forever Marilyn in Shanzai, China
Fn2 hyperallergic.com

Some Like It Hot
Fn1 Billy Wilder's glittering masterpiece has topped BBC cultures 100 greatest comedy pg1. Nicholas Barber explains why https:www.bbc.com/culture/article/20170817
Fn2 Film Excerpt. 'Some Like it Hot' A.H. Weile, Books March 30, 1959
Fn3 https:/www.rogerebert.com/reviews. SomeLikeitHot.1959
Fn4 https:/www.bytimes.com/2020/06/02/WeStill-LikeItHot.A.O.Scott.and Manohla Dhargis

More About Marilyn
Fn1 Homolog.US
Ibid pg14

Rotten Tomatoes
Fn2 Rotten Tomatoes.com
Fn3 Professional Beauty Newsletter.Joanna Sterkowicz, August 23, 2021

Marilyn Monroe Relationships (2d time with Einstein, etc.)
Fn1 Homolog.US
Fn2 According to his attorney, Morris Engel

VII. Marilyn Monroe Relationships
Fn1 Homolog.US
Fn2 According to his attorney, Morris Engel

Fn3 https:/www.thebash.com/search/marilynmonroe-imperson-ator-newjersey
Fn4 Ibid: VIEW PROFILE
Fn5 Ibid: VIEW PROFILE
Fn6 (after the Korean War) https://discoverwalks.com/blog/unit-ed-states/top-10-shocking-facts-about-marilynmonroe
Fn7 ibid. pg. 4-5
Fn8 ibid. pg. 9
Fn9 ibid. pg. 13

Los Angeles Times
Fn1 From the Archives: Marilyn Monroe dies, Pills Blamed. Howard Hertel and Don Nef. The Los Angeles Times.

"The Psychoanalyst" (the first time)
Fn1 Britannica Dictionary definition of Psychoanalyst.

The Funeral of Marilyn Monroe
Fn1 http:// www.marilynmonroe.ca/camera/about/facts/funeral.html

Carrie Fisher Footnotes
Fn1 https://www.latimes.com/local/lanow/la-me-in-carrie-fisher-au-topsy-report-20170619-story.html
Fn2 https://cnn.com/2016/12/23/entertainment/carrie-fisher-cardi-ac-arrest
Fn3 https://www.mirror.co.uk/3am/celebrity-elizabeth-taylor's red-hot-affair. pg4

Fn1 https://www.biography.com/news/carrie-fisher-debbie-reyn-olds-relationship.pg2
Fn2 ibid, pg2
Fn3 ibid, pg2

Fn4 ibid, pg2
Fn5 ibid, pg2
Fn6 ibid, pg2
Fn7 ibid, pg2-3
Fn8 ibid, pg3
Fn9 ibid, pg3
Fn10 ibid, pg3
Fn11ibid, pg3
Fn12 Carrie Fisher Opens Up About Star Wars, the Gold Bikini, And her on-set Affair.
https://www.npr.org/transcripts/503580112

Anthony Bourdain Footnotes
Fn1 Anthony Bourdain, Wikipedia, pg2
Fn2 ibid, page 8
Fn3 ibid, pg11
Fn4 ibid, pg2
Fn5 ibid, pg10
Fn6 ibid, pg6
Fn7 ibid, pg7
Fn8 ibid, p9.1
Fn9 ibid, pg1
Fn10 ibid, pg4
Fn11 ibid, pg4
Fn12 ibid, p95

Appendix

Hippocampal neurochemistry, neuromorphometry, and verbal memory in non-demented older adults, Zimmerman et. al., n.neurology,org/content/70/18/1594.

In this study, forty-eight older adults had smaller hippocampal volumes and abnormal levels of certain metabolites in them. They had significantly impaired verbal memory function. Another word for diminishment in size of a body organ or part of an organ is "atrophy."

One important biochemical molecule operative in the hippocampi is N-acetyl aspartate. It plays an important role in memory. Creatine is a waste product. Patients with clinical depression were studied with a complex imaging procedure[42] and in-depth psychological testing.[43] Hippocampal N-acetyl aspartate ratio was abnormal (NAA/C), with significantly diminished NAA to creatine. The findings showed that both lower hippocampal N-acetyl aspartate predicted decreased, impaired memory ability.

<u>Additional metabolic abnormalities in the hippocampi in Major Depression</u>. Again, employing Magnetic resonance spectroscopy.[44]

Two additional biochemical molecules were found to be deficient in the hippocampi in clinically depressed patients, lactate and choline.

---

42 4-T MRI, proton magnetic resonance spectroscopy.
43 Cued Selective Reminding Test – Immediate Recall, Wechsler Memory Scale-Revised; Trail Making Test Parts A&B.
44 Hippocampal neurometabolite changes in depression treatment: A magnetic resonance-spectroscopy study. Psychiatry Res. 2012 MARCIANO. 31: 2011 (3) 206-13.

Lactate serves as a fuel in the neurons (brain cells) to provide energy for normal neuronal metabolism. It also maintains upkeep for axons (the main "cables" leaving the body of the neuron, making contact with other neurons) for normal interneuron communication. It is important in the consolidation of memories (i.e., so "remembering" is possible). Choline plays a role in the formation of acetylcholine, an important neurotransmitter in memory functions. A neurotransmitter permits neurons to communicate via their synapses (or connecting bodies), in which the neurotransmitter travels from one neuron to the next, again essential for interneuron communication.

The discussion of these three biomolecular deficiencies in the hippocampi of people with major depressive disorder is *not* all-inclusive.

The researchers concluded: "In light of our findings and previous studies results, we hypothesize that mitochondrial dysfunction leading to predominantly anaerobic gycolysis in connection with the intracellular signaling pathways disturbances and decreased astrocytic function/number might subsequently lead to deceased brain neuroplasticity in depression. These mechanisms could be positively influenced by antidepressant treatment with selective serotonin or norepinephrine reuptake inhibitors with potential effects on untimely neuronal aging in depression."

Translation:

Mitochondria: Small, energy-producing bodies inside the cells (i.e., neurons). They are, so to speak, the "power plants" in the cell. Dysfunction means reduced energy supplies for the cell.

Anaerobic glycolysis: One-way cells (neurons) change sugar (glucose) into lactate (lactic acid) for energy. It is less efficient than aerobic glycolysis in the presence of normal oxygen supplies. Impaired neurons have insufficient oxygen.[45]

Intracellular signaling pathways_(disturbance): Signaling systems within a cell by which there is communication from the inside to the outer membrane, or within the cell, which regulates cell growth,

---

45 Medianenet.com/mitochondrial-disease/article.htm.

proliferation, and cellular processes necessary for survival. Obviously, disturbances of it will be detrimental to a neuron.

Neuroplasticity (decreased). The ability of networks of neurons to adopt, change, reorganize, and make new connections in response to the requirement to function healthily as an individual in adapting to life's demands and stresses. It is obvious that the greater the impairment in neuroplasticity, the greater will be symptoms and disabilities.

Study: Variations in myo-inositol in frontal limbic regions and clinical response to electroconvulsive therapy in Major Depression.[46]

Myo-inositol is a type of sugar which provides energy to the brain. It plays an important role in the neuron (brain cell), transmitting signals from receptors on the outside of the cell membrane to the inside in order to permit important neuronal biological activities.

Frontal-limb regions: Important brain regions regulating focused attention, relaxation, and changes in or shifting of mood states, emotional processing, and decision-making. In major depression and bipolar disorder, there is decreased activity.[47]

Dorsal-medial-anterior cingulate cortex (DMACC): A series of interconnected brain regions that could be a part of a broader anxiety circuit, playing a role in the integration of "threat information" (obviously from the environment), which then "orchestrates" a response: "through synchronized activity with distant brain regions" then resulting in selected cognitions (thoughts) and motor control (behavior).

Description of study. Individuals in a major depressive episode (clinically displaying the symptoms) had been shown to have reduced levels of myo-inositol in the frontal-limbic brain region. Fifty patients received a course of ECT. They were matched to controls who did not receive ECT. Brain scans using magnetic resonance spectroscopy demonstrated the ECT-treated patients showed increasing levels of

46   Njau, Stephanie et.al. 10.106 J. J psychires 2016.05.012.
47   Common and distinct abnormal frontal-limbic system. https://pubmed.ncbl.nlm.nih.gov/20069426.

myo-inositol in the DMACC and hippocampus paralleling symptomatic improvement in their depressive illnesses.

Note: There was no suggestion that deep unconscious conflicts were resolved with the treatment, but instead, a particular biochemical in specific brain regions was significantly elevated and enhanced. The controls who did not receive ECT did not demonstrate enhanced myo-inositol or symptomatic improvement. The authors postulate symptomatic improvement was associated with "neurogenesis," the birth of new neurons (the opposite of hyperapoptosis).

Study: "Effect of Electroconvulsive therapy on Striatal-Morphometry in Major Depressive Disorder. [48]

An important circuit in the brain is the limbic-cortical-striatal-pallidal-thalamic circuit.) These different brain areas operate together to regulate the mood-state and emotional regulation. Patients with major depression have reduced size and volume of striatal and pallidal structures, key components of the circuit.

The striatum is part of the basal ganglia, which are large nuclei (concentrations of neurons) below the cortex (surface of the brain). The basal ganglia play a role in movement and the control of movement. It serves as an "intermediary" between cortical, amygdala, and striatal circuits "for cognition, action, motivation and reinforcement. It is a key locus for convergence of brain circuits involved in reward, learning, hedonics, and motivation."[49]

Question: Are the deep emotional conflicts hooked into the basal ganglia? The basal ganglia sounds very important! The pallidum is a part of the basal ganglia which sends signals via its fibers (axons of neurons) to other structures, including projections to the thalamic nuclei, the anterior and lateral nuclei, and the medial dorsal nuclei. It is a central component of the reward system and contains the brain's

48   Wade, Benjamin S.C., et al. Neuro-psychopharmacology. 2016 Sept. 41(10); 2481-91. Doi: 10.1038/npp. 2016, 48.
49   Basal ganglia. Wikipedia//https://en.wikipedia.org/wiki/Basal.ganglia.

pleasure centers regulating motivation, behavior, and emotions. It is also involved in addiction.

Fifty-three patients with clinical (major) depression underwent a course of ECT treatment. The control group was thirty-three subjects without a history of major depression. An imaging technique, structural MRI, was used to measure size and volume of striatal and palladial structures before, during and after ECT treatment. The depressed patients had smaller striatal and palladial volumes than the controls. After completion of the course of ECT, dorsal and ventral striatum and palladial volumes were significantly increased. This did not occur in the controls. One would postulate that with treatment, increased neurogenesis (the opposite of apoptosis, characterized by the birth of new neurons) accounted for the improved size metrics.

Another study, "Depression is associated with hippocampal volume loss in adults with HIV.[50]

Is HIV-AIDS a "mental" problem? Is major depression a "physical" problem? No, it's the other way around! But they both shrink the hippocampi. But one does that by purely "mental" processes (evidently deeply buried unconscious conflicts can shrink the hippocampi).

Recap: people with major depression have smaller hippocampi than so-called normal people, the result of an atrophy process fueled by hyperapoptosis. People with HIV-AIDS have smaller hippocampi as a result of low CD4 immune cells, independent of depression. No one would assume people with HIV-AIDS are therefore "mental cases" because they have smaller hippocampi vs. clinically depressed individuals, even though they don't have major depression. Psychiatry allows people to believe deep emotional conflicts account for the smaller (atrophying) hippocampi in the "mental cases."

It is just common sense not to attribute that cause in people with HIV-AIDS; for them, it's obviously a "physical" abnormality. In the unfortunate individuals with HIV-AIDS and comorbid major depression, the effect on the process of atrophy of the hippocampi is cumulative.

---

50   Bronshteyn, M. et. al. PMD 340 89-726 PMCID: PMC8288081, DOL: 10.1002/ hbm 25451.

Milton Keynes UK
Ingram Content Group UK Ltd.
UKHW050252280324
440097UK00006B/38